D0209375

University Branch

NO LONGER PROPERTY OF
SEATTLE PUBLIC LIBRARY

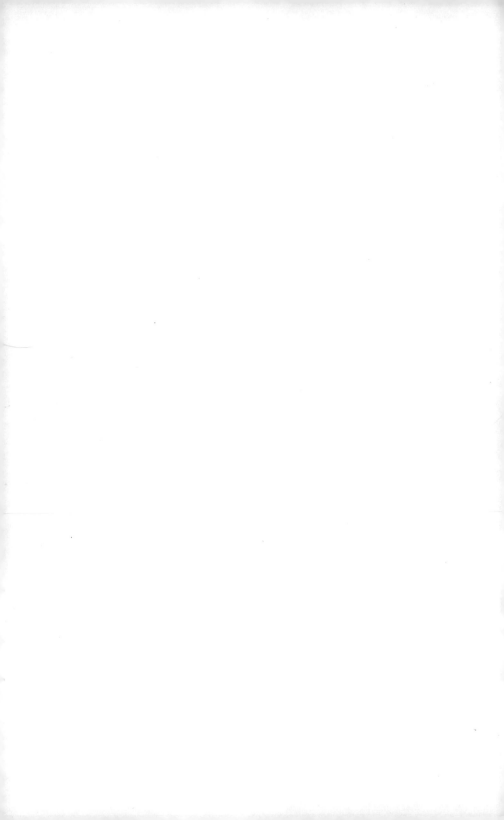

PALEO DOG

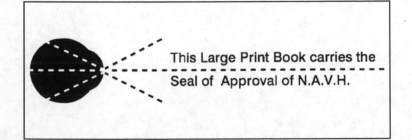

This Large Print Book carries the
Seal of Approval of N.A.V.H.

PALEO DOG

GIVE YOUR BEST FRIEND A LONG LIFE, HEALTHY WEIGHT, AND FREEDOM FROM ILLNESS BY NURTURING HIS INNER WOLF

JEAN HOFVE, DVM, AND CELESTE YARNALL, PHD

THORNDIKE PRESS

A part of Gale, Cengage Learning

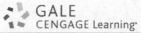

GALE
CENGAGE Learning®

Farmington Hills, Mich • San Francisco • New York • Waterville, Maine
Meriden, Conn • Mason, Ohio • Chicago

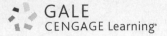
GALE
CENGAGE Learning®

Copyright © 2014 by Jean Hofve, DVM, and Celeste Yarnall,PhD.
Illustrations by Michael Gellatly.
Chapter opener and sidebar art by iStock. by Getty Images.
Thorndike Press, a part of Gale, Cengage Learning.

ALL RIGHTS RESERVED
Mention of specific companies, organizations, or authorities in this book does not imply endorsement by the author or publisher, nor does mention of specific companies, organizations, or authorities imply that they endorse this book, its author, or the publisher.
Internet addresses and telephone numbers given in this book were accurate at the time it went to press.
Thorndike Press® Large Print Health, Home & Learning.
The text of this Large Print edition is unabridged.
Other aspects of the book may vary from the original edition.
Set in 16 pt. Plantin.

LIBRARY OF CONGRESS CATALOGING-IN-PUBLICATION DATA

Hofve, Jean, author.
 Paleo dog : give your best friend a long life, healthy weight, and freedom from illness by nurturing his inner wolf / by Jean Hofve, DVM, and Celeste Yarnall, PhD. — Large print edition.
  pages cm. — (Thorndike Press large print health, home & learning)
 Reprint of: Emmaus, Pennsylvania : Rodale, [2014].
 Include bibliographical references.
 ISBN 978-1-4104-7309-7 (hardcover) — ISBN 1-4104-7309-0 (hardcover)
 1. Dogs—Nutrition. 2. Dogs—Food. 3. Dogs—Health. 4. Large type books.
I. Yarnall, Celeste, 1944– author. II. Title.
SF427.4.H68 2014b
636.7—dc23   2014024566

Published in 2014 by arrangement with Rodale Press, Inc.

Printed in Mexico
1 2 3 4 5 6 7 18 17 16 15 14

To Willy, my best canine pal,
whose gift to me was
a great love for all dogs!
— *Jean Hofve, DVM*

To Nazim, my beloved husband,
whose love and support
gives my heart wings.
— *Celeste Yarnall, PhD*

CONTENTS

PREFACE

Pretend with us, for a moment, that we are making a movie about our modern dogs' ancient ancestors, wild wolves, to show what life was truly like for them.

PALEO DOG ~ The Movie

FADE IN:

EXT. SNOW-COVERED LANDSCAPE — DUSK

We SEE on the horizon a pack of healthy TIMBER WOLVES, running at full tilt, chasing their intended prey, a YOUNG LONE DEER. We HEAR their heaving panting as they run. STEAM rises from their open mouths as they dart through the heavy snow. Suddenly — WHAM — it's over. The DEER is down. The FEEDING begins.

9

CLOSE ON ALPHA WOLF AND DEER

ALPHA WOLF, with fangs bared, digs into the deer's rump and bolts down huge pieces of meat. The ALPHA FEMALE WOLF gulps down a few pounds of rump meat, then moves around and opens the carcass just behind the ribs. She eats a portion of the liver and several strips of fat from the mesenteric membrane. The rumen is dragged away by a subordinate wolf; he rips it open and shakes it to let the contents spill out onto the ground, then lies down to chew on the muscular organ. The large intestine is dragged away and subsequently ignored. Small bones are eaten; larger bones, including the long bones of the legs, skull, and vertebrae, are stripped of meat and cartilage; they are chewed on but not consumed. When the pack moves on, there is little left besides hair, hide, and bones. This PACK will sleep on full stomachs and live to see another day.

SLOW DISSOLVE — A MODERN GERMAN SHEPHERD DOG at his DINNER BOWL:

We see our proud wolves' descendant,

today's selectively bred, pedigreed GER-
MAN SHEPHERD DOG looking down at
his bowl of KIBBLE, which is sitting in a
wire rack. For a moment, there is a flash
of confusion, as though he doesn't quite
understand what to do. His deep brown
eyes look full into the CAMERA, trying to
tell us something important. He sighs, low-
ers his head, and eats.

FADE OUT

Everything about the wolves in our hypo-
thetical movie script shows us that canines
are meant to hunt and kill their dinner. And
they eat it raw, not cooked, kibbled, bagged,
or canned, and not in cute shapes or fun
colors.

The wolf and its wild relatives (wild dogs,
jackals, coyotes, and foxes) are completely
dependent on their ability to chase prey, kill
it, and devour it with jaws and teeth designed and conditioned to do so. It is the
hunt, kill, and eating of the carcass — bones
and all — that keeps them in top condition.

In *Paleo Dog,* we will share with you how
to safely integrate the best of the ancestral
dogs' lifestyle into the daily regime of your
modern dog and help you navigate the

promises and pitfalls of 21st-century living and modern veterinary medicine.

INTRODUCTION

There was a time in human history when we operated more like our animal kin, a time when we humans and wolves were more alike than different. Survival by co-operation was a given, so we traveled in packs, and wolves did, too. We often competed for the same prey animals.

Our collective basic needs were taken care of more efficiently by cooperative living. "Survival of the fittest" isn't really historically accurate; it was more like survival of the strongest and best organized — communities or packs succeeded by working together.

In this book, we'll travel back in time to the Paleo period to see how those lifestyle principles can work in our lives today. This will help us re-create a Paleo lifestyle that will be just right for your dog and the current stage of his life and health.

We grew up in the 1950s, which is often

13

thought of as a more innocent time (although not quite prehistoric!). We believed in our doctors, and we only had one, who made house calls when we were sick. Veterinarians made house calls as well, especially to farms and ranches. Doctors encouraged chicken soup, and veterinarians used more natural treatments, including herbs and special elixirs, for our animal companions, while also incorporating miraculous new drugs like antibiotics.

Back then, we believed our doctors and veterinarians had the answers to everything. We all operated from a belief system that simply made it easy for us to turn over our health and well-being to these specialists, who themselves learned from scientists teaching in respected institutions. But then everything got more and more complex, as did the systems that were employed by the medical experts we trusted. New medical models and standards of care were developed. Vaccinations became the preventive care of choice, and we accepted this without question.

The problem is that the new specialists didn't deserve the trust we placed in them.

Modern medicine does too much for too little gain. There is an obsession about naming the disease, or localizing the lesion, or finding out *exactly* what the problem is, whether or not such knowledge will have any practical consequence. Doctors perform extreme diagnostics, and if they're lucky, they can triumphantly put a name to a condition. This extreme pursuit of a precise diagnosis seems to stem from the ancient superstition that naming a thing gives you power over it.

What we've come to realize today is that veterinary medicine has gone down the same path as human medicine. There are lots of machines and special medical toys, but in the end, they likely won't help your dog. You can get a diagnosis that doesn't mean anything in terms of fixing the problem. If you are going to use a diagnostic tool (especially a very expensive one), you want to make sure that the information it gives you will make a difference in how you treat the dog. Does it matter what kind of liver disease or what the genesis of the kidney disease or the diabetes is if the treatment is going to be the same? A dog with diabetes will always need insulin, whether the diabetes occurred because of infection, diet, or autoimmune disease from vaccines.

Many modern diseases, including obesity, heart disease, and depression, are caused by lifestyle — in particular, a sedentary lifestyle. We're stuck in our desk chairs and couches, and our dogs are stuck, too. There's a growing movement and desire to return to the way our ancestors lived: outdoors, active, and self-sufficient. This isn't to say we should ditch civilization 100 percent, but what if we shifted just 5 percent of the way toward a more Paleo lifestyle? That's what we're trying to do here: help you and your dog get back to your roots, eat fresh whole foods, run around more often, and get plenty of fresh air and sunshine.

It may sound easy enough, but we're up against some big guns: the American Medical Association, the American Veterinary Medical Association, and of course the Food and Drug Administration. We were taught to trust these organizations and look to them to protect us for everything health related. What a mistake! (Of course, there has always been a fringe group of so-called health nuts and tree huggers who rebelled — fellow oldies will remember Jack La-Lanne, Adelle Davis, Rachel Carson, and many others. But as life got more and more complex and specialized, our information sources dwindled to sound bites, corporate-controlled news reports, and commercial and paid advertisements, all of which had and still have huge financial motivation to put out the fires that the health nuts occasionally start up.)

Since we were babies, we've all been consistently pushed and brainwashed — with any occasional spark of Paleo-instinctive thinking stifled — and driven to turn over our nutritional and medical needs to others. When it comes to feeding ourselves and our animals, the old adage "let thy food be thy medicine" has been forgotten and replaced with time-saving devices and shortcuts like microwave ovens and prepackaged food. We've traded our natural diet for fast food. But in the Paleo period, for both man and wolf, the only "fast food" was that which ran, swam, or flew away!

We choose what is convenient as opposed to what is healthy and healing. And the fast-food paradigm, with its gluten-heavy grains, chemicals, additives, and preservatives, is killing us all in record numbers.

Do you remember the slogan "better living through chemistry"? One by one, chemicals have replaced natural substances as cleaning solutions and problem solvers, and now, even food is being replaced by genetically modified organisms (GMOs). Something as basic as our water supply is being polluted by toxic chemicals like chlorine and additives such as fluoride.

Our dogs' food is also born from convenience. Most of the big pet food companies are offshoots of mega-corporations: Nestlé Purina (Dog Chow, ProPlan, Beneful), Procter and Gamble (Iams, Eukanuba, Natura), Colgate-Palmolive (Hill's), Mars (Pedigree, Royal Canin, Nutro), Del Monte (Kibbles 'n Bits, Milo's Kitchen, Nature's Recipe). These companies have convinced us that we can no longer trust ourselves to know how to feed a dog (or that it's too time-consuming). All you have to do is open a bag of kibble or a can of "fresh meat"! Your dog will come running and not only enjoy this meal but also shower you with grateful, slobbery kisses.

Sure, the big pet food companies have done a lot of research; they have scientific *data*! But if you look at the history of commercial pet food, you see that there have been many stumbles and U-turns, and many pets have paid the ultimate price with their health and their lives.

A few decades ago, pet food manufacturers started substituting more and more plants and grains for meat. After all, meat was expensive. Many veterinary nutritionists say a calorie is a calorie and ingredients don't matter, so the companies figured that

18

corn gluten meal would be just as good ¿ rib-eye steak and that they could make ¿ bigger profit. Dogs will gobble it up, and the stockholders will be thrilled!

Let's take another example: choline, a member of the extended B-vitamin family. When pets don't get enough choline, their cognitive function declines and they become senile. A good friend of ours, Shawn Messonnier, DVM, discovered that supplementing choline could actually reverse these problems. Now, choline is a required ingredient in pet food, but the required minimum is intended only to prevent outright deficiency, not to provide an optimal level. Choline and the other B vitamins are found in abundance in animal products, particularly liver. But they're fragile and easily destroyed by heat. Canned and dry pet foods are supplemented, but is it enough — and enough for what? To keep them alive, but not healthy? Of course, rather than put more actual nutrition in pet foods, it's more profitable to create a drug to combat senility in dogs. So if you go to your veterinarian, you can get the drug, but you probably won't be told that a vitamin supplement might do just as well.

Is that how we want to treat our dogs? Is it okay to say, "They have the mechanisms to make up for what we're not giving them, so don't worry about it"?

Pet food must meet certain standards and protocols set by an organization called the Association of American Feed Control Officials (AAFCO). It does provide Nutrient Profiles that list 36 specific nutrients — vitamins, minerals, amino acids, and fats — but it still hasn't decided how much of the omega-3 fatty acids eicosapentaenoic acid (EPA) and docosahexaenoic acid (DHA) should be in pet food. New profiles are in the works (the last ones are more than 30 years old), but they won't list a minimum requirement for adult dogs. Therefore, budget-conscious pet food makers won't put them in, and dogs will go without, as usual. (Even in dog foods that do include EPA and DHA, the amounts are not enough to balance out the vast overage of omega-6s, which tend to promote inflammation, or really to do much of anything.)

In the wild, dogs would have gotten EPA and DHA from their grass-eating prey. But now their "prey" comes from the grocery store, and it's corn-fed or corn-finished, and corn does not provide the raw materials that herbivores need to make healthy omega-3s. On top of all that, American corn is genetically modified, soaked in pesticides, and grown in deficient soils. Dog food is not providing the nutrients that our dogs would get in nature. There's definitely something wrong with this picture!

So, we will revisit the Paleo lifestyle and understand more clearly what "Paleo" really means. We will take what works and bring it back to the present day. You will see and decide for yourself how much of it resonates for you and your dog.

The Paleo lifestyle movement offers us an alternative to what we find today in most pet food aisles and veterinary clinics. *Paleo Dog* is an exciting option for those who realize that Mother Nature did and does indeed know best.

However, to implement the Paleo Dog Lifestyle, we need to start with a checkup of our own belief system and to reexamine some of the ideas that have become so much a part of our lives today, such as the germ theories and zealous warnings about raw natural foods like meat and bones. Instead of being driven by fear, we need to revisit the harmony and balance of life and our internal, external, and planetary ecology.

To understand and implement this healthy, beneficial lifestyle, we need to reset our belief systems in an independent, mature, and thoughtful way. We hope *Paleo Dog* will help you do just that.

■ ■ ■ ■

PART I
THE PALEO DOG

■ ■ ■ ■

CHAPTER 1
WHAT IS A PALEO DOG?

BANG!

That's how it all started.

Of course, it took a few billion years for stars and planets to form and for life to evolve from stardust into the vast complexity we have today on Earth.

The earliest life forms, simple bacteria, set the stage for everything that followed: more complex bacteria, algae, fungi, insects, fish, birds, and mammals — including us humans and our dogs.

The first bacteria were very basic, no-frills, single-celled organisms. The next step was to get together, since a community functions better than just one individual. One speculated result was the formation of more-complex bacteria containing "organelles," little mini-organs that took on certain specific functions, such as respiration, elimination, and reproduction. Those organelles may have started as other free-living bacteria that became incorporated within the new cells. These new and improved bacteria were so successful that they became the template for all life forms to follow.

The Paleolithic period, or Stone Age, began about 2.5 million years ago, as the earliest humanoid ancestors began using crude stone tools, and lasted until about 10,000 years ago, when agriculture began. Fully developed *Homo sapiens* may have entered the scene as early as 1.4 million years ago.[1] During the Paleo period, humans lived as hunter-gatherers, eating what they could kill, scavenge, or harvest. Also during that time — probably around 400,000 years ago — humans learned to control fire and use it for cooking (although jambalaya and beef bourguignon weren't on the menu quite yet).

The endpoint of the Paleo era was when early humans, the hunter-gatherers, figured out how to make food stay in one place — and agriculture was born. Once people settled down in groups that no longer wandered around looking for something to eat, civilization, as we know it, emerged.

But looking around at what civilization has become — we're fatter and sicker than ever before — people have started looking back at our evolutionary diet and rethinking how far away our modern diet is from those basic beginnings.

The Paleolithic, or Paleo, diet (also called the Stone Age or Caveman diet) has become a popular concept for modern people. Surely it's not just wistfulness for days gone by; after all, those days were pretty harsh! No, it's appealing because folks think of our most distant ancestors as thinner and healthier (not to mention hairier — maybe good news for those suffering from male pattern baldness!). Since the Paleo diet first took off in 2007, its popularity has skyrocketed, as more and more people return to this ancient way of eating.

Proponents of the human Paleo diet suggest that people should eat a diet similar to that eaten by their great-great-great-great-great-great — well, you get the idea — grandparents: fresh animal-based foods, and the rest from plants. This diet is thought to have been high in protein (20 to 35 percent of calories), high in fat (30 to 50 percent), and low in carbohydrates (20 to 40 percent, composed mostly of complex carbohydrates). Fortunately, the conveniences of modern life make it possible to hunt and gather right there in the grocery store.

The wolf ancestors of today's dogs began

associating with humans about 130,000 years ago, according to DNA evidence. They were hanging around the hunters, picking up scraps, for a very long time before people settled down to farm.

Canines, although classified in the order Carnivora (meat-eaters), more typically live as "facultative" or "opportunistic" omnivores. This means that, given the opportunity, they'll eat just about anything! But the canine family in general is designed to eat primarily prey animals. That sort of diet contains more protein and fat, and much less plant material, than the early human diet. The nutrient ratios for dogs would be closer to 45 to 55 percent protein, 40 to 45 percent fat, and less than 10 percent carbohydrates.

But the Paleo Dog Program is about much more than diet. Our dogs' ancestors were physically and mentally active, lived in the fresh air and sunshine, and had a rich social life with both humans and their own kind. They weren't vaccinated, they weren't neutered, and they weren't medicated. On occasion, they also had to deal with some serious problems: food shortages, infectious diseases, injuries, and parasites.

Nevertheless, the canine species not only survived but also thrived! We can learn a great deal from their example, and we can bring the best of both worlds — Stone Age and modern — together to create the healthiest lives for our dogs today.

THEN AND NOW

There are more than 78 million dogs living in American households today. About 85 percent of them eat commercial dog food.[2] At least half of them are overweight or obese.[3] More than three-quarters of them have significant dental disease by the age of 3.[4] Cancer kills 42 percent of all dogs and 50 percent of the dogs more than 10 years of age.[5] *None* of these problems plagued dogs in prehistoric times.

The typical dog's life today goes something like this:

1. Born of mixed-breed heritage
2. Dewormed, vaccinated, and re-homed before the age of 3 months
3. Eats one brand of dry "kibble" dog food for most of his life
4. Neutered between 2 and 6 months of age
5. Spends 8 to 10 hours a day alone at home
6. Is confined mostly to a fenced yard, or goes on occasional walks

7. Gets revaccinated annually, has flea-protection applied monthly, and gets a heartworm pill every month
8. Gets less exercise with increasing age
9. Dies between 10 to 13 years of age, most likely from cancer

As it turns out, wild wolves also live about 10 to 13 years, despite their hazardous lifestyle (up to 17 years in captivity).[6] This suggests that, despite loud and frequent claims that "better nutrition" (i.e., commercial dog food) and better health care (i.e., lots of vaccinations and drugs) have greatly extended dogs' life span, it hasn't actually increased by much, if at all. The main difference in life span among today's dogs is primarily genetic and size-related: Small dogs live longer, and big dogs die younger; mixed-breed mutts tend to be healthier, while purebred dogs often have hereditary health problems that can cut their lives short.

EARLY WARNING SIGNS OF INTERNAL IMBALANCE

Ninety-eight percent of dog guardians consider their dogs healthy. Unfortunately, most of them are wrong, simply because they do not recognize the early signs of ill health; nor do most veterinarians.

There are many signs or characteristics of internal imbalance — harbingers of overt disease — that most people would consider "normal."[7] But while they may be common and average, they are *not* normal. As our dogs become healthier, we find that these "normal" things go away. In young, healthy-appearing animals, the "normal" issues listed below may be the only indication that trouble is brewing.

A recent study of 45 dogs age 9 or older found that 80 percent of them had at least one health problem that was previously recognized.[8] The mean number of problems was seven to eight per dog. Issues found in the exams included heart murmurs and arrhythmias, dental disease, ear infections, liver disease, arthritis, and several cancerous tumors. It's essential to have a thorough health screening of your dog at least once a year, especially as he gets older.

Subtle Signs of Imbalance

Skin
Doggy smell
Fleas

Dry, oily, or dull coat
Excessive shedding
Ear problems-waxy, oily, itchy
Recurrent mites
Eye discharge
Excessive tearing
Matter in corner of eyes
Raised third eyelid
Discoloration or spots on or in the eye

Behavior
Fears (loud noises, thunder, people, life)
Too timid
Too rough or aggressive (even at play)
Too hard to train
Barks too much or too long
Suspicious nature
Bites when petted too long
Hysteria when restrained
Clumsy
Lazy
Overlicking or sucking on objects

Digestive
Bad breath
Tartar accumulation
Periodontal disease
Loss of teeth
Poor appetite
Craving or eating weird things (rubber

bands, plastic, dirt, paper, poop, rock
Excessive thirst
Redness along gum line
Frequent vomiting
Mucus-coated stools
Diarrhea with any change of diet
Obesity
Anal gland problems

Musculoskeletal
Stiff when getting up
Early hip dysplasia
Tires easily in hot or cold weather
Cannot go up or down steps
Fragile, thickened, or distorted claws
Claws painful or sensitive to trim

Temperature
Low-grade fever (normal for healthy dogs
  is 100 to 101.5°F)

Age and Reproduction
Diminished life span (large breeds should
  live up to 17 years, giant breeds up to
  12)
Difficulty conceiving easily, delivering
  normally, and passes along "genetic
  breed" problems

OBESITY

It's estimated that more than 55 percent of American dogs are overweight or obese, so there's a pretty good chance that your dog, or a dog you know, is one of them.[9]

Sorry, but we have to be brutally honest with you: Fat dogs are not cute, or cuddly, or even comfortable — they are sick. Excess weight reduces life expectancy and increases a dog's risk for many serious health problems, including (but definitely not limited to) the following:

- Joint disease (including arthritis)
- Heart disease
- Hypertension (high blood pressure)
- Respiratory problems
- Asthma
- Pancreatitis
- Diabetes
- Liver disease
- Skin and coat problems
- Anesthetic complications
- Impaired immune function
- Reduced life expectancy
- Cancer

While there may not be a *known causative* link between diet, obesity, and specific diseases, there is certainly a dietary effect in

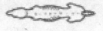

VERY THIN Body Score = 1

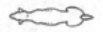

THIN Body Score = 3

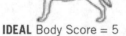

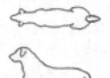

IDEAL Body Score = 5

OVERWEIGHT Body Score = 7

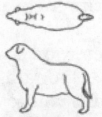

OBESE Body Score = 9

35

the risk for and management of those diseases.[10]

Is your dog too fat? A dog is overweight at a body condition score of 6, and obese at a score over 8. Ideally, you should be able to easily feel your dog's ribs; from the side, the belly should tuck up, and from the top, there should be a discernible waist.

Based on research, the "ideal" score for body condition is about 4.5, a little less than the ideal on the chart. Most people would consider that thin, or even too thin. However, a longevity study conducted on 48 paired Labrador Retrievers showed that life expectancy was significantly longer in the leaner animals. In addition, age-related conditions such as arthritis developed much later in thin dogs.[11]

Did you see the movie *Super Size Me,* about a guy who decided to eat at McDonald's for breakfast, lunch, and dinner every day for a month? After a couple of weeks, his doctors begged him to stop because they could see the devastating impact his experiment was having on his health.[12]

Commercial pet food has a lot more in common with McDonald's food than its manufacturers want you to know (including the fact that spoiled and discarded food and waste grease from McDonald's may actually be an ingredient in your dog's dry food).[13] Fast food is cheap, full of carbs, and loaded with fat — but the carbs (especially sugar) and fat make it taste good, and may even make it addicting![14]

Adipose (fat) cells are quite active. They produce hormones and other chemical messengers, including inflammatory proteins. The chronic low-grade inflammation and oxidative stress that goes along with obesity causes or contributes to arthritis, heart disease, and other inflammatory conditions[15] — even cancer.[16]

Veterinary nutritionists rely on three basic concepts:

1. To lose weight, burn more energy than you eat.
2. A calorie is a calorie.
3. Ingredients don't matter, only nutrients matter.

However, if these simple ideas were the whole story, neither we nor our dog companions would be facing the current obesity crisis. Individual genetics may play a larger role in canine obesity than in human obesity; for both, however, the biggest culprit is diet — though not in the way veterinary nutritionists typically frame it.

"Energy" is just another word for "calories" — a calorie is a measurement of energy. Protein and carbohydrate each provide 4 calories per gram of food; fat contains 9 calories per gram. This makes fat more "energy dense." Therefore, veterinary nutritionists who formulate pet food substitute carbohydrates for fat. It's a nice bonus for pet food makers that carbs are also the cheapest ingredient.

However, ever since "low-fat" foods were introduced, the Western world has gotten fatter. Recent research makes it abundantly clear that fat is not the problem; carbohydrates are — and in particular, highly digestible carbohydrates. (Fiber is also a carbohydrate, but it is indigestible and does not contribute to the calorie count.)

Modern research makes it clear that a calorie may be a calorie in the lab, but in a living organism, other factors affect metabolism, obesity, and weight loss. Whether calories come from carbs, proteins, or fats appears to have a significant impact on health.[17]

Weight management or "light" dog foods, which research has shown vary tremendously in calories, are not reliable.[18] And simply substituting a different kind of kibble

isn't the healthiest way to lose we
your dog, either. Kibble is energy-
that is, there are a lot of calories
tiny packages.

While most veterinary nutritionists are still stuck in "low-fat" mode, it's actually simple carbohydrates that are the problem. Starches, like those found in corn and potatoes, rapidly increase blood sugar and have deleterious effects on insulin metabolism.[19] Research shows that a high-protein, low-carbohydrate diet is the safest and most effective weight-loss program for dogs. It helps them lose more body fat and retain more lean muscle mass.[20]

The ideal diet is also low in energy density. Diet density can be lowered by increasing either indigestible fiber, water, or both.[21]

To illustrate the effect of dietary water, think about potato chips versus mashed potatoes. Potato chips are high-density: almost no moisture and a lot of fat. In contrast, mashed potatoes (without butter or gravy!) are lower in density. They contain a lot of moisture. Most folks can eat a lot of potato chips before they feel full, but mashed potatoes tend to fill them up in a hurry. A high-moisture diet will help your dog feel full on fewer calories.

Additionally, high dietary protein has been

own to increase satiety; this means that ubjects stayed satisfied longer after eating a high-protein meal than after consuming a meal with other formulations.[22]

Research shows that nearly half of dogs who lost weight regained it, largely because they didn't stay on their diets — or more accurately, their guardians did not keep them on their diets. Only you have the power to solve this problem for your dog.

INFLAMMATION AND AGING

One thing that science has discovered is that inflammation is at the root of many diseases, as well as the process of aging. Aging and disease occur because of free radical damage, also called oxidative stress. We need to look at this phenomenon in more detail to understand how and why the Paleo Dog Lifestyle is so important.

It's a fundamental truth that all animals live and die at the cellular level. If our cells aren't healthy, then it's a quick trip to cellular dysfunction, organ malfunction, disease, and death.

All cells need energy to do their jobs, as well as to maintain and repair themselves. Tiny "engines" within cells burn oxygen and fuel to produce energy, which in the body is a molecule called adenosine triph-

40

osphate (ATP). These little engines are called mitochondria, and they produce massive amounts of ATP every day. As the mitochondria burn fuel, just like a car engine does, not only is energy created but other by-products are created as well. We used to think that these other molecules were waste products, similar to the CO_2 and ozone from gasoline-burning engines. But it turns out that the body makes these by-products, these extra molecules, on purpose. In fact, these "signaling molecules" are one of the body's most important methods of communication. Cell signaling is how all the trillions of cells in the body talk to one another, work together, and act as a cohesive unit. It's absolutely fundamental to life.

Some of these molecules are oxygen-free radicals, or simply, free radicals. You may have heard of these molecules as the "bad guys" in terms of inflammation and aging. However, these molecules aren't all bad. The immune system uses free radicals to attack and kill invading viruses and other pathogens.

However, things like inflammation, stress, vaccination, genetically modified foods, junk food, electromagnetic radiation, pesticides, and air pollution, along with the normal wear and tear of living, can cause production of excess, unbalanced free radicals. It's the accumulation of these unbalanced free radicals that leads to the condition called oxidative stress.

While a certain amount of free radicals is necessary for the body to function, *excess* free radicals are like loose cannons. They can damage enzymes, fats, DNA, and proteins. Accumulated free radical damage over time is associated with diseases of aging, such as arthritis, cognitive dysfunction, and heart disease. Many cancers are also thought to have their origins in oxidative damage to DNA.

Since free radical formation is a normal process, the body has a natural regulatory system in place: endogenous (native) antioxidants scavenge and dismantle excess free radicals. Vitamins C and E are probably the best-known antioxidants, but the body also makes "master" antioxidants (glutathione peroxidase; superoxide dismutase, or SOD; and catalase), which work efficiently and effectively to neutralize free radicals whenever and wherever they get out of control.

However, while dogs do produce their own endogenous antioxidants, they simply can't produce enough to combat the extraordinary stresses of modern life — things that their ancestors were never exposed to,

like noisy, crowded city streets. These stre
sors increase free radicals, which in turn
lead to damaged cells, organs, and tissues.

So, is there any way to prevent these
damaging effects?

Giving your pet antioxidant supplements
is one way to boost the immune system and
protect against free radical damage. However, exogenous antioxidant supplements
have only limited effects in the body. The
fact that they seem to work quite well
indicates that animals have so much oxidative stress and free radical damage that even
a teeny tiny increase in antioxidant activity
has a big effect!

Endogenous antioxidants are enzymes,
which are specialized proteins that catalyze
(speed up) chemical reactions without being changed or harmed by the reaction.
These master antioxidants are speed de-
mons; they can neutralize millions of free
radicals per second. Because they are enzymes, they just keep on going. Endogenous
antioxidants also can move in and out of
cells.

Plant-based exogenous antioxidants are
big and slow. And because they aren't
enzymes, they can neutralize only one free
radical before they're done. Antioxidants
from food or supplements are absorbed

from the intestines into the blood, but that's as far as they go. Now, there's plenty of work for them to do right there in the bloodstream, but they can't protect cells from damage to DNA or other structures inside the cell, like mitochondria.

Healthy puppies come into the world with a full supply of mitochondria and signaling molecules; their cells are working at top efficiency. However, starting around puberty, cells produce fewer mitochondria, and the number of mitochondria continues to decline as the years pass. In fact, free radicals themselves actually damage the mitochondria. Fewer or damaged mitochondria means less energy, as well as fewer signaling molecules. When that happens, lots of free radicals build up, oxidative damage progresses, and the end result is aging.

The Paleo Dog Program incorporates many methods of reducing oxidative stress and slowing the aging process. First, we take care of diet — the food eaten by most dogs today actually causes increased free radical production, as well as a buildup of toxins that inhibit cellular function.

Exercise and stress reduction are two of the big guns of free radical control, so these are a significant part of the Paleo Dog Lifestyle.

The Paleo Diet for Dogs

Like its counterpart for humans (which excludes dairy products, cereals and grains, beans, and all salty or processed foods), the Paleo Dog Diet is a natural diet. By this, we mean one that is appropriate to the species and that contains the fewest possible "unnatural" processed, synthetic, and chemical ingredients. The basic Paleo Dog Diet features raw meat and is grain-free and gluten-free.

The diet includes:

- Bones (including poultry, organ meat, and eggs)
- Fresh, nonstarchy vegetables and fruits
- Omega-3 marine oil
- Probiotics and digestive enzymes
- Vitamins, minerals, and supplements

Hundreds of holistic veterinarians recommend a homemade, raw-meat diet for their patients. Raw food is, of course, what wild canines eat — and have eaten for millions of years. We've seen and heard literally hundreds of stories about pets' skin disease, allergies, autoimmune disease, seizures, dental problems, cancer, and dozens of other conditions — from annoying to deadly — being resolved solely or primarily by a switch to a raw-meat based diet. It really is common sense to feed our dogs what they were designed to eat.

While dog biscuits have been around for a long time, it's only in the past 60 years or so that commercially produced dog food became popular and turned into the sole diet for so many dogs.

Once humans learned to control fire, they likely cooked most or all of their meat, and newly domesticated dogs may have shared cooked scraps. However, they also scavenged the parts of the carcass that the humans did not want, and those were eaten raw. They may also have continued to hunt on their own now and then, and always consumed their prey raw. Dogs ate this way for thousands of years.

As civilization advanced, humans moved across the globe, and their dogs went with them. As humans learned to eat the foods they found in their new environments, their dogs also adapted to the local diet. In the frozen north, Huskies and Malamutes doing heavy work lived on fish, game, and blubber. In Central America, petite Chihuahuas got along on leftover grains and beans from their human families, plus whatever mice or rats they could catch. European Spaniels and Retrievers ate offal from game birds as well as bread and vegetables.[23]

As civilization continued to develop, dog breeds became more refined, but their health started to suffer — not only because of the faulty genetics of inbreeding and line breeding but also from the gradual departure from their ancestral diet.

One of the most common objections to using a "wild" or natural diet for today's pampered pooch is "Aren't our domestic dogs too different from their wild ancestors?"

Some will go so far as to say that because humans have tinkered with dogs' genetics so much — creating dozens and dozens of different sizes, breeds, and temperaments — dogs now *need* human-made food!

Recent research shows that dogs have indeed adapted to increased amounts of starch in their diets. Dogs' DNA has actually changed so that they are better able to digest starch and utilize glucose than their exclusively carnivorous wolf ancestors were.[24] But are those changes significant? More important, is this good news or bad news for dogs?

It is definitely good news for the pet food industry. Since dogs *can* derive nutritional value from many kinds of foods, manufacturers take advantage of this to substitute more and more nonmeat ingredients for the natural meat-based, high-protein diet our dogs are meant to eat. But, as they say, just because you *can* do a thing doesn't mean you *should.*

Let's take a trip down the dog food aisle at the local grocery, discount, or pet store to see what the real problem might be. Here's what you'll see if you read a few labels.

Popular veterinarian-recommended dry dog food: Chicken, *pea protein concentrate, potato starch, dried potato,* chicken meal, chicken fat, *dried beet pulp, flaxseed,* chicken liver flavor, *powdered cellulose . . .*

Popular weight-control dry dog food: Turkey, *brewers rice, corn gluten meal,* poultry by-product meal, *corn bran, whole grain corn, whole grain wheat, oat meal,* natural flavors, beef tallow . . .

Popular grocery-/discount-store-brand dry dog food: *Ground whole corn,* meat and bone meal, *corn gluten meal,* animal fat (preserved with BHA/BHT), *wheat mill run, ground wheat,* natural poultry flavor, *wheat flour,* salt, potassium chloride, caramel color, vegetable oil (a source of linoleic acid), *rice, wheat gluten . . .*

Wait a minute — didn't we just say that dogs are carnivores? So what are ingredients like peas, potatoes, corn, wheat, rice, and oats doing in dog food? They're replacing more expensive animal-based ingredients, so the manufacturer makes a bigger profit.

There's a good reason why diet is the foundation of the Paleo Dog Program: Most serious health problems in dogs have a dietary component. Some are actually caused by diet, and all are affected by it. These medical problems can damage your dog's quality of life and your wallet, since many of them are expensive to diagnose and to treat. In the chart on page 50, do you see any similarities between nutrition-related diseases and the most common reasons dogs visit the veterinarian?

Other canine diseases that are caused or exacerbated by diet include obesity, developmental orthopedic disease, progressive renal disease, insulin resistance, Cushing's disease, hypertension, exercise intolerance, respiratory distress, heart disease, reproductive disorders, pancreatitis, and cancer. Even apparent behavior problems such as irritability, fearfulness, aggression, jealousy, excessive grooming, and elimination issues may have a nutritional component. After all, when you don't feel good, your behavior is likely to suffer, too.

Top 10 Reasons for Veterinary Visits	Nutrition-Related Diseases
Ear infections	Food allergies
Skin allergies	Skin allergies
Pyoderma (hot spots)	Skin and coat problems
Stomach upsets (not the same as "upset stomach")	Chronic vomiting
Intestinal inflammation/ diarrhea	Inflammatory bowel disease/diarrhea
Bladder diseases	Urinary tract inflammation
Eye infections	Decreased immune function
Arthritis	Arthritis
Hypothyroidism	Hypothyroidism
Sprains	Joint and orthopedic disease

No matter what medicines, supplements, or treatments you give your dog, none of them is as important to overall health as diet. An animal cannot heal its body if its nutritional needs remain unfilled.

As we've seen already, dogs are — genetically and physiologically — 99.8 percent identical to wolves. All free-roaming members of the canine family are carnivorous hunters, and we believe that our dogs are better off following as similar a regime as possible. However, there are also cautionary tales of *Salmonella, Toxoplasma,* and other organisms contaminating raw meat that can make your dog — and you — very sick. A raw diet is not for every pet, especially those with medical conditions. As the ratings folks say, "Discretion is advised."

We will be discussing diet and nutrition in detail later, so stay tuned! In the meantime, let's go back to the common sense we once had, which seems so absent today, and feed our dogs the way they should be fed, as well as help them live the lifestyle that made the original Paleo Dogs so robust and durable.

THE PALEO DOG LIFESTYLE

The Paleo Dog Program isn't just about diet. It's also about the dog's whole lifestyle. Many factors contribute to degeneration, aging, and the tragically short life span of so many of our dog breeds. Nobody needs to remind us that we're all aging at a very rapid rate; our bodies are breaking down sooner, and we have a host of lifestyle diseases that are largely preventable: the so-called diseases of civilization, or diseases of affluence. Our dogs are paying the price for that, too.

But what are we doing wrong? Most dogs are missing out not only on a healthy diet but also on the whole spectrum of activities and life habits that early Paleo Dogs had but that we seem to have lost.

Let's be realistic, though. In order for dogs to get along today, they need to be trained, and they need to be spayed or neutered (primarily because too many people are irresponsible about canine overpopulation). Both we and our dogs must make certain accommodations in order to live in the modern world. The Paleo Dog Program is about doing the things we can to make up for the detriments of modern life.

The Paleo Dog Lifestyle is a return to canine roots. While Paleo-promoting humans have focused exclusively on nutrition, the Paleo Dog Program is a truly *holistic* change in lifestyle that encompasses physical, emotional, and mental well-being. It relies on four main principles:

1. Good nutrition (the Paleo Dog Diet)
2. Appropriate veterinary care — annual exam, fewer vaccines, better dental health

3. Sunshine, exercise, and play
4. Respect, love, and communication

People have an infinite array of choices when it comes to diet, environment, and lifestyle, but our dogs are subject to the choices we make. They have to eat what we give them to eat, exercise when we decide they should, and socialize only when we allow them to do so. When we invite dogs into our homes, we are completely responsible for their quality of life. They can't grab the car keys and head out for a burger. They can't decide to go to the gym on Saturday. Most dogs can't even decide when and where they'd prefer to poop or pee! What they eat, where they sleep, and how they spend their days are all under our control.

The concepts in *Paleo Dog* are for people who want to create the best possible lives for their dogs. And by the way, following these precepts will very likely influence and improve your health and life, too!

Tips to Get Started

We highly recommend that you keep a journal for each animal in your care. This way you can track each step along the

---

way, such as what you fed the dog and when, how the dog's appetite was, the amount of exercise or other activities, and so on, as well as remedies and treatments and their effect. That way, if your dog has been making progress but plateaus or backslides, you can easily go back to the previous step. And you'll also be able to see how much progress your dog is making toward truly optimal health. As you start to incorporate *Paleo Dog* principles, we encourage you to proceed step-by-step and not try to get everything accomplished in 24 hours!

CHAPTER 2
HISTORY OF THE DOG

As we learned in Chapter 1, dogs and humans have been friends for about 130,000 years. But the canine family was around long before that.

The modern dog is descended from a branch of carnivorous mammals that shared the distinction of having four carnassial teeth adapted for tearing apart flesh. Examining fossilized remains reveals how these teeth evolved from their earliest function of crushing and chewing to the strong, sharp teeth of true meat-eaters. The first carnivores (prevalent 38 to 54 million years ago) belonged to a diverse genus called *Miacis* — small weasel-like mammals. As the size and number of herbivore animals increased, so did the size and number of carnivores.

Many believe that the dog's closest relatives lived in North America and belonged to the now-extinct genus *Hesperocyon* (26 to 38 million years ago), the first true canid to appear after the canine and feline branches of the order Carnivora diverged. *Cynodictis* followed (19 million years ago); this successful carnivore belonged to the genus *Amphicyon* and developed independently around the world.

By the Myocene period (about 12 million years ago), the genus *Tomarctus* appeared on the North American scene, with the beginnings of the modern dog's dentition. At this time, approximately 42 different genera of canines had developed. But by 2 million years ago, the 42 genera of canines had consolidated into the 9 genera we have today.[1] *Canis,* the largest genus, contains the "true dogs": wolves, jackals, coyotes, dingoes, and dogs. These species are all more closely related to one another than to the next largest group, *Vulpes* — the true foxes. (Hyenas, as doglike as they appear, are not in the canine family at all; in fact, they are more closely related to cats.)

THE FIRST PALEO DOG

After 40 million years of evolution, an international team of scientists identified what they believe to be the world's first real dog, a large-toothed, big dog that lived 33,000 years ago in Altai in Central Eurasia.[2] This was the original Paleo Dog, which subsisted on a diet of horse, musk ox, and reindeer. The second oldest dog, from about 14,000 years ago, was found in Russia. However, wolf bones have been found together with human bones that date back more than 100,000 years, suggesting that a peaceful coexistence, if not friendship, was blossoming well before humans took an active hand in the process.

It has been proven by modern DNA testing that the sole ancestor of today's domestic dog is the wolf. As pack animals, the first wolves to engage in a relationship with humans already had the social skills and personality traits that would ultimately make them humankind's best friend. Thus, the most important aspect of early Paleo Dogs — the vital ingredient that put them on the long road to domestication — was their behavior, and specifically, their behavior with respect to humans.

Recent research shows a significant difference in the way wolf cubs and dog puppies experience their environment. While both animals' senses (smell, hearing, and sight) develop at the same rate, wolf cubs start actively exploring at just 1 week of age — 2 weeks earlier than puppies — while they are still deaf and blind. The cubs startle more easily as well. This suggests that the prime socialization period for wolves is earlier and shorter than that for dogs.[3]

We don't know what the first contact between wolves and humans was. Undoubtedly, human groups and wolf packs loosely coexisted for many generations before their paths merged. Wolves that ventured closest to people might, over generations, have become tame enough to touch. It's likely that Paleo humans knew where the wolves' dens were; they could have taken unattended or orphaned cubs to raise by hand. It wouldn't take long to figure out that the friendliest cubs were the best bet. These naturally tamer pups must have been the ancestors of the modern dog.

We know that this is the most likely scenario because the same circumstances have been re-created in modern times. In 1959, Russian geneticist Dmitri Belyaev speculated that the key to the domestication of animals was a trait that he called tamability. He also suspected that this tame behavior was linked to physical characteristics; that is, the DNA that coded for tamability (genotype) would lead to the behaviors and looks that characterize the domestic dog (phenotype). Belyaev founded the Institute of Cytology and Genetics in Siberia and began an experiment with silver foxes — bred and raised in fur farms — that continues today.

Farm foxes are somewhat tamer than wild, free-roaming foxes, but they are by no means people-friendly; they have little contact with humans other than being fed and having their cages cleaned.

Belyaev's team tested fox pups for tameness beginning at 1 month of age and continuing once per month thereafter, by offering food by hand and attempting to pet each pup. At 6 or 7 months of age, foxes were separated into three groups: tamest, neutral (neither friendly nor aggressive), or wildest. Interestingly, females were much more likely to display tame behavior — 20 percent of females, but no more than 5 percent of males, made the cut. The tamest foxes were bred with each other, and the tamest pups were selected from each litter to continue the experiment. After 30 to 35 generations, the foxes in the tamest group were not only docile and friendly pets, displaying behaviors such as whining and competing for human attention, but had taken on some distinctive physical features as well: piebald coats (patches of white fur), a curled tail, and rounder ears. They also experienced physiological changes in their digestive, nervous, and reproductive systems.[4]

Canine domestication may have occurred more than once, with many and far-flung groups of wolves. Wandering groups of people and semi-domesticated wolves may have subsequently crossed paths with others, increasing the genetic diversity as their wolf-dogs interbred.[5]

As human beings shifted from being nomadic hunter-gatherers to farmers living in communities, the wolf stayed with them, and in doing so, changed its ways. Selective breeding began, and so developed the domestic dog.

THE AGRICULTURAL REVOLUTION

Humanity's dietary habits had remained the same for *Homo sapiens'* entire existence to that point: They ate the meat they could kill or scavenge and the fruit, vegetables, and nuts they could gather. But then came the agricultural revolution, and grain quickly assumed a prominent position in the diet.

Humans genetically adapted to their new high-starch diet by increasing the number of copies of the gene for amylase, an enzyme that breaks down carbohydrates.[6] More gene copies means more of this enzyme is produced. This enables humans to get a jump on starch digestion with amylase in the saliva that gets mixed into the food by chewing — rather than waiting until the food passes through the stomach and enters the intestines, where the pancreas contributes the biggest dose of digestive enzymes, including amylase.[7]

In their evolution from wolves, dogs also increased the production of amylase, but only in the pancreas; they still lack salivary amylase. Depending on diet, humans express from 4 to 16 copies of the salivary amylase gene; dogs express from 4 to 30 copies of pancreatic amylase.[8]

DEVELOPMENT OF THE CANINE FAMILY

Nine thousand generations later, members of the family Canidae share many of the same characteristics:

- Distinctive body language that enables them to communicate with one another — for example, how the tail is positioned and how its hairs move.
- A large brain capacity that has allowed wolves to evolve into social hunters. The pack relationship has enabled them to successfully hunt and bring down much larger animals than any

single wolf could alone, and has provided safer conditions for rearing pups. (However, domestic dogs' brains are 10 to 30 percent smaller than wolves' brains.)[9]

- Excellent hearing and exquisitely sensitive noses — all the better to sense prey at long distances.
- Long skulls supporting strong cheek muscles to pierce and hold on to prey, kill it, and devour it.
- Front limbs with a "locked" radius, and ulna bones that cannot rotate, providing them with stability when running.
- Semirigid hind legs that provide them with excellent endurance.
- Compact feet with tough but sensitive pads that can take the impact of running full speed over any terrain, yet also cushion the feet for near silence while stalking prey.
- A scent-marking gland on the dorsal surface of the tail, which allows them to leave a scent whenever or wherever they raise or wag their tails. This is variably expressed in different dogs — in some it's unnoticeable; in others, it's extremely active.

Our own Paleo ancestors must have realized that a tamed wolf could be useful for hunting, guarding, and other tasks, and begun selecting for specific physical and behavioral traits.[10]

Here are the four breed groups based on DNA evidence:

- Dogs of Asian and African origin
- Herding dogs and sight hounds
- Modern hunting dogs such as terriers, hounds, and retrievers
- Large Mastiff-type dogs

In addition, 14 breeds have been identified by DNA analysis as "ancient" or "basal." All other breeds are thought to derive from them:

- Afghan Hound
- Akita
- Alaskan Malamute
- Basenji
- Canaan
- Chow Chow
- Dingo
- Finnish Spitz
- New Guinea Singing Dog
- Saluki
- Samoyed

- Shar-Pei
- Shiba Inu
- Siberian Husky

THE MODERN DOG

There are now hundreds of pedigreed, man-made breeds, each with a distinctive look and behavioral characteristics and recognized by one or more registries, such as the American Kennel Club (AKC). Each breed has an official standard, which causes us to reflect on how far they have come from those first wild dogs that our ancestors domesticated. Of course, the majority of dogs today are not pedigreed but are mixed breeds of uncertain parentage.

Parent breed clubs for seven groups of dogs have mapped out standards that cover how the dogs are to be judged in the show ring. Judging criteria include general appearance, temperament, conformation (physical structure and traits), gait, size, and penalizing faults.

The seven AKC classifications are broken down as follows (with a few samples of breeds within those categories):[11]

1. **Herding group** (*Collie, Shetland Sheepdog, Border Collie, Briard, and Old English Sheepdog*). Early hu-

man beings captured wild animals, corralled them, and used them for agriculture and livestock farming. They did not wish to have these animals run away and be eaten by predators, so they devised a way to protect them. The early sheepdogs were bred and trained for such a purpose.

2. **Working group** *(German Shepherd Dog, Alaskan Malamute, Siberian Husky, Saint Bernard, Leonberger, Mastiff).* The working dogs have an innate ability to warn people of impending danger (for example, a trespassing enemy). Thus, the guard dog was born. Other examples are military and police dogs, sled dogs, lifesaving dogs, fighting dogs, and service dogs.

3. **Sporting group** *(American Cocker Spaniel, Irish Setter, Labrador Retriever, Weimaraner).* The sporting dogs are known for their incredible sense of smell. They can alert people to the whereabouts of birds that have been shot down. They are also capable of retrieving them. Many are strong swimmers and will retrieve from the water.

4. **Hound group** *(Afghan, Borzoi, Greyhound, Basset, Beagle).* Hounds are classified in two groups: sight hounds and scent hounds. The sight hounds are spotters who can see far away and chase their prey until it drops from exhaustion. These dogs can run up to 35 miles per hour. Racing Greyhounds are an example of this group's speed and agility. Scent hounds, like Bloodhounds, are used extensively by the police to search for drugs and bombs.

5. **Terrier group** *(Fox Terrier, Airedale, Kerry Blue Terrier, Welsh Terrier, Jack Russell Terrier).* The word *terrier* comes from the Latin *terra,* meaning "soil." These dogs love to dig and were used to hunt prey that hides in burrows.

6. **Toy group** *(Pekingese, Chihuahua, Maltese, Papillon, Bichon Frise, Pug, Pomeranian).* As the name suggests, toy dogs are the smallest of all. Many were bred to literally be lap dogs. There are some hounds, sporting dogs, and terriers that fall into the toy group because of their small

size. People love them as companions, and they are just plain cute. They live nicely in small quarters, such as city apartments.

7. **Nonsporting group** *(Keeshond, Dalmatian, Chow Chow, Poodle, Shar-Pei, Lhasa Apso, Schnauzer).* This group encompasses dogs who may be suited for specific work, but are not related to dogs in other groups. They are found in circus acts, are used as ratters, and make excellent guard dogs.

The history of dogs is inextricably woven together with our human story, and our bonds have grown closer with each generation — from being wolves on the fringe to their relatively new status as our best friends (and even de facto children). It took until the end of the 20th century for us to acknowledge that dogs are capable of so much more than just physical jobs. Their love and companionship have impacted our society as well as our individual lives. Through their unconditional love and loyalty, they teach us to be more humane. We owe it to them to ensure they live a full and healthy life alongside us.

PART II
WHY YOUR DOG
SHOULD GO PALEO

■ ■ ■ ■

CHAPTER 3
BENEFITS OF BEING
A PALEO DOG

Today, modern dogs fed conventionally on commercial food may be smelled before being seen. You know these dogs because they greet you at your friend's home, or you see them on the street. Their human companions, of course, love them and think that they are the most wonderful dogs in the world. And they believe you should think so, too.

But as you smile and greet your friend, the dog's foul breath will practically knock you over. The dog's human family may be completely acclimated to the odor, but to your unprepared nose, the smell coming from the dog's decaying teeth and infected gums is repulsive. This condition is appropriately dubbed "mouth rot" by Aussie vets. (We have more polite terms, such as *periodontitis,* for dog dental disease here in the United States.)

Averting your head from the dog's mouth,

you may notice another smell: that warm, musty, doggie odor emanating from every pore. When the dog comes up to you for a welcome pat and a big hello, tail wagging nonstop, the condition of his fur may not be so inviting to your touch — although you give the dog a pat or two for politeness's sake. Maybe the fur is greasy-looking, or dry and flaky, but it's clear to you this dog's coat is in very poor condition.

Now that you are up very close and personal with this friendly, seemingly happy dog, you might also notice — as you give him a little scratch on his head — that there is another smell wafting up from his ears. You see a dark, waxy buildup on the inner ear flap. Perhaps the corners of his eyes have a wad of dark crud, affectionately dubbed "eye boogies." There might even be some redness or excessive tears in the eyes as well. His lower eyelid might droop a little, so you can see hundreds of tiny blood vessels in and under it.

If you visit for long enough with this dog, you may be treated to yet another aroma: doggie flatulence!

Your friend has now invited you to stroll along with them. It is quite obvious from the gaseous odor you have just inhaled that this dog has business to attend to very soon!

As the dog pulls him along, your friend is poised, plastic bag at the ready, to attend to the inevitable cleanup that must be done. You continue along, and — at last — the dog selects just the right spot. He circles a few times and deposits a steamy pile of an excessively large volume of stool. Its foul odor almost makes you lose your balance.

Did you notice on this walkabout that there was a bit of weakness or wobbliness in the dog's hind legs? Even though he is definitely carrying too much body fat around his middle (just like many people we know!), his hindquarters look kind of caved in on the sides. You politely ask how old this dog is, and the answer astounds you: only 5 years old.

Having rid himself of his load of stool, the dog now seems more cheerful and ready to limp along. As you proceed together, he sneezes several times when he stops to smell the flowers or grass. Periodically, he also plops his butt on the ground and vigorously scratches at his ears.

If you ask your friend what the dog eats, the answer will almost certainly be this or that brand of dry kibble. But then your friend will add those magical buzzwords after the brand name, "It's all natural!" You also learn that it was recommended especially for this dog by a trusted veterinarian.

At this point, you are very happy that this is not *your* dog, and you are determined to help your own dog avoid these problems. You have seen this happen among your friends' dogs far too often! You start wondering, what could be the common denominator that causes these all too frequently observed symptoms to appear?

Then you wonder how your friends feel when they encounter your dog at your home or on a walk. Your dog can't be *this* bad, right?

THE SUBTLE SIGNS OF DISEASE

All of the issues you noticed with your friend's dog, as well as the many other subtle, early signs of disease we listed in Chapter 1, are common annoyances and complaints to veterinarians the world over. Most often, these dogs do get adequate veterinary care, and may even be eating expensive prescription diets for conditions such as allergies, digestive problems, arthritis, heart disease, or urinary system issues. They may even be receiving one or more medications for an array of chronic health complaints.

Many of these chronic and persistent problems start in the mouth. Periodontal

disease is the most common problem v[ ]
narians see, and a completely prevent[ ]
problem. It begins with the normal bacte...
that live in the mouth. These bacteria
secrete substances that create a protective
biofilm (protective for the bacteria, that is
— not for the dog!), which rapidly develops
into plaque. The minerals in saliva harden
the plaque into tartar (calculus). Tartar on
the tooth can easily be seen, but that's not
where the real problem is; this gunk gets
under the gums as well.

Bacteria, too, thrive in the natural pocket
between the tooth and the gum. Their secretions cause trouble here as well: The immune system responds, and inflammation
and damage to the tooth's supporting ligaments, and eventually the bone itself, are
the result. Ultimately, the tooth will loosen
and fall out. But that isn't the worst problem.

Because of the inflammation and tissue
damage in the mouth, bacteria that normally
live on the surface gain access to the bloodstream, where they are carried throughout
the body. Studies of dogs have shown that
bacteria associated with periodontal disease
cause microscopic changes in the heart,
liver, and kidneys that can lead to serious
disease in those organs. [1]

Of course, the entire process of inflammation and decay is painful to the dog. However, because these changes occur gradually, most dogs accommodate to the discomfort and may never show overt signs of pain. Their breath will smell pretty bad, but until it becomes truly foul, many people just don't think to have their veterinarian check it out. Now, you might ask, "Don't all dogs have bad breath?" No! They don't, they shouldn't, and it's not normal. Average, maybe, but not normal.

Back in the 1940s, when commercial dry food gained huge popularity, some veterinarians observed that pets' dental health seemed to be declining.[2] While pet food makers have had to create new foods to fix the problems their other foods were causing, feeding raw meaty bones as little as once a week has long been known to prevent dental calculus.[3]

Tens of thousands of dog guardians, breeders, handlers, and trainers are now feeding a species-specific Paleo-type diet to their dogs and seeing the end of many nagging problems. Here are some of the benefits that they report and that we have seen for ourselves, both personally and clinically.

PALEO DOG HEALTH BENEFITS

There are many benefits to be gained from the Paleo Dog Diet and Lifestyle.

Cleaner teeth, healthier gums, fresher breath, and less periodontal disease. The varied textures in the Paleo Dog Diet will reduce plaque deposits. Raw meaty bones, ground into the food or sized appropriately for your dog, work like a natural toothbrush, scrubbing, scraping, massaging, stimulating, and even flossing the teeth.

Easier dental care. Those stressful times at the veterinary clinic for dental work under anesthesia won't occur as often, which decreases the risk of complications for your dog.

Improved oral health for at-risk breeds. Small and brachycephalic breeds, such as Pugs, Pekingese, Boxers, Bulldogs, Shih Tzus, and Chihuahuas, are at high risk for periodontal disease because of overcrowding and malocclusion of their teeth. However, they are still carnivores and will benefit from smaller bones such as raw chicken necks.

Better digestion. Physiologically, your dog's gastric juices start working to get ready for the meal even before it arrives in his stomach. When you place the food before him, he begins to eat by working his jaws and teeth on the fleshy meat, with its sinew and bones. This takes time, causes him to eat slowly, and offers him enjoyment. More gastric juices are secreted so that the food can be digested properly.

Improved stool quality. Firmer, smaller stools with less odor are observed soon after conversion to the Paleo Dog Diet. Stools may contain powdery white material from bones, which is normal. They degrade into the soil if deposited there. Poop patrol becomes a lot less unpleasant (though it will probably never be a fun job). And there's another bonus: no more flatulence!

Shinier, healthier skin and coat. Say goodbye to doggie odor and dandruff, and hello to a healthy, glossy coat and normal skin. You'll notice decreased shedding and less dryness, greasiness, and flakiness. Dandruff stops, and hot spots start healing. Skin and coat improvements are often rapid (2 to 3 weeks) and dramatic.

Resolution of allergy symptoms. Cooking denatures (distorts) proteins; the two rounds of high-heat processing that dry food undergoes make it more likely to trigger intolerances and allergies. Raw meat is far more digestible, and its normal proteins are better tolerated by the immune system.

Improved muscle strength and stability.

The shredding, tearing, and bone-crushing activity that come with the Paleo Dog Diet also help to build up strength in the jaws, neck, back, and shoulder muscles. The Paleo Dog Lifestyle's increased activity strengthens skeletal and heart muscles, enhances cardiovascular function, and improves balance and flexibility.

Weight normalization. With the Paleo Dog Program, your dog will attain and maintain a healthy weight. Exercise improves strength and balance, which means fewer musculoskeletal problems. It also helps increase metabolic rate, which will make your dog feel better and will make maintaining an optimal weight much easier.

Better performance. Working dogs, show dogs, agility dogs, and other high-performance dogs feel better because they are well nourished, and their bodies aren't burdened by the many additives in commercial pet food. They have more energy and spunk, and therefore perform better.

Less inflammation. Pasture-raised and 100 percent grass-fed meat, poultry, dairy, and eggs are leaner and contain healthier fats than corn-fed, factory-farmed products. These natural foods also contain more antioxidants, such as vitamin E, beta-carotene, and vitamin C, and have less cholesterol (though your dog doesn't care about that!).[4] Another benefit is that they don't contain traces of added growth hormones, antibiotics, or other drugs. There are fewer calories in grass-fed meat because it is lower in fat. It also contains two to four times more vitamin E and omega-3 fatty acids than meat from grain-fed animals. Omega-3s have anti-inflammatory effects, while omega-6s mostly contribute to ongoing inflammation. However, one beneficial omega-6 found in meat and dairy products is conjugated linoleic acid (CLA), which is anti-inflammatory. Evidence suggests that the particular form of omega-6 found in animal products can prevent cancer.[5] The good form of CLA is higher in grass-fed animals.[6]

Antiaging. The omega-3s found in higher quantities in pasture-fed meat and eggs have many benefits, including antiaging potential. Omega-3s may prevent the shortening of telomeres, the "caps" on the ends of chromosomes. The shortening of telomeres over time is thought to be involved in degeneration and aging.

Increased stamina. Even older dogs experience energy levels that you may not have seen in years. You and your dog may find that you take longer walks because of his increased stamina, which benefits both of you!

Lower food bills. While there are some unavoidable start-up costs when you first convert your dog to the Paleo Dog Diet, analyses have found that ongoing costs are quite comparable to feeding him premium dog food. A *Bark* magazine article reports that the cost of homemade dog food is "still less than the cost of feeding high-end commercial food."[7] Ways to reduce costs include buying ingredients wholesale, watching for sales on meat, and working with your local butcher to obtain meat scraps, organ meat, and meaty bones at a lower cost.

More love. The loving connection and bond between you and your dog will strengthen as your dog observes the daily ritual of food preparation. This loving act on your part becomes a very real ingredient in the diet, as your dog anticipates and looks forward to what you have prepared for him, thus strengthening the human-animal bond and the interspecies communication. You both benefit from this exchange on an emotional and spiritual level. People also report that their relationship improves as their dogs feel more comfortable in their skin. And, of course, the increase in longevity will give you and your dog more healthy years together.

HONORING THE ECOLOGY
OF OUR PLANET

The environment and ecology of our entire planet benefit when its life-forms eat their biologically appropriate natural diet. This is especially true of carnivores, as they perform many vital functions. For example, large carnivores like wolves and bears regulate the number of herbivores like deer and elk by taking fawns, and they keep herds healthy by preying on the old, sick, and injured. Canines also play an ecologically important role as scavengers.

Studies of the wolves reintroduced to Yellowstone National Park in 1995 have shown that their presence has had wide-ranging effects. They changed the behavior of the park's elk, which quit hanging around in thick foliage and now stay in open areas where they can see predators coming. These wolves initially killed 50 percent of the coyotes in the greater Yellowstone ecosystem, which increased the survival of pronghorns, which wolves themselves do not hunt.[8] The return of the wolf has even impacted plant growth. Willows, cottonwoods, and other trees are growing normally for the first time in decades because the elk are out in the open instead of browsing on young shoots.[9]

Both canines and felines have litters of multiple pups and kits, while prey like bighorn sheep, deer, elk, and bison have one or two calves (three at most) at once. But only the strongest and smartest survive, and nature maintains a system of balance between the eaters and the eaten.

At the other end of the scale, smaller carnivores are pitted against smaller prey like rabbits and rodents, which can have a new litter every few weeks. Fortunately, it takes a lot of mice to fill up a coyote, bobcat, or fox, so their numbers are also kept in check by predation.

In studies known as Pottenger's Cats, Dr. Francis Pottenger conducted long-term feeding experiments on a large group of cats, which he fed combinations of raw or cooked meat, and raw or pasteurized milk, and noted their effects on the cats' own health and that of their progeny. Raw-fed cats and their offspring were much healthier. The feeding experiments eventually came to a close, and the cats were removed from their pens. It was subsequently observed that weeds had begun to grow in the empty pens. However, there were noticeable differences in their size and health: The weeds were bigger and healthier in the pens where the cats had been fed a raw meat diet, but sparse and spindly in pens of cats that had been fed a cooked food diet.[10]

The Pottenger team embarked on a new series of experiments based on these observations. They planted navy beans and fertilized them with noncomposted excreta from cats fed either a raw meat or cooked meat diet, and left a control plot unfertilized. At first, the beans showed little difference, but as they grew, plants in the raw meat plots were the biggest and healthiest, plants in the unfertilized plots came in second, and those in the cooked meat plots were pale and spindly. Next, beans harvested from the first generation were planted and fertilized with composted manure from cats fed raw meat, cooked meat, raw milk, or pasteurized milk, along with some planted in an untreated control plot. Similar results were obtained, and it was also noted that the root growth of the raw-meat fertilized plants was far more extensive and sturdy than that of the others.

The next year, another experiment was conducted with plants grown in composted manure from cats fed raw meat, cooked meat, raw milk, or pasteurized milk, and in an unfertilized control plot. Again, not only was plant growth best in the raw meat plot, but also the beans harvested were larger, more uniform in size and shape, and more nutritious than the others.

Clearly, the cats fed naturally had naturally fertilized the soil. When cats were fed cooked, lifeless food, not only were they less healthy, but also their wastes were so devoid of nutrients, and perhaps even toxic, that plant growth was inhibited.

Healthful eating has a ripple effect on local ecology, but multiply that times billions of animals, and it is clearly affecting the entire ecology of our planet.

Pottenger demonstrated the connection that all life shares, and the way our ecosystems are dependent on one another. His studies show the reciprocal relationship that plants, animals, and humans have with Earth. We are all interdependent and essential parts of the web of life.

Our soil is critically important in this web. It must be renewed and vitalized by the bacteria, fungi, and all other life that teem in it — all of which were here long before mammals. Plants have ancient and symbiotic relationships with the organisms that live in the soil.

When animals eat biologically appropriate

food and their waste is returned to the soil, it nourishes that earth, so the cycle of life continues in harmony. However, when animals do not eat their natural, species-appropriate diet (and instead eat processed, preserved dog kibble), this natural cycle is interrupted — much like when chemical fertilizers are used instead of organic compost, synthetic pesticides are poured on crops, and toxic manure from corn-fed feedlot cows pollutes groundwater.

These careless acts by humans lead to the death of earthworms and other life-forms that inhabit the terrain. The soil itself becomes dead, unable to support life without the "artificial life support" of chemical fertilizers.[11]

Today, most cities require "proper" disposal of dog feces; unfortunately, their definition of "proper" usually means poop-filled plastic bags piling up in a landfill. Because we now have so many dogs in numbers that a natural environment would not support, some have suggested that simply having a dog is ecologically disastrous. We disagree. When dogs are fed appropriately, their fecal volume is smaller and safe to compost.

Pottenger's experiments offer us a wealth of information that has been all but forgotten by modern scientists. Perhaps we can do our small part by allowing what goes into our dogs to come out as a benefit to the whole cascade of life that endlessly renews itself. The health of all of our animals affects the health of our soil, thereby affecting seeds, plants, animals — all of us — and our planet as well.

Visit the Vet Less Often

The biggest advantage of the Paleo Dog Diet and Lifestyle Program is the resolution of health problems and far fewer chronic complaints. Degenerative disease processes and conditions will usually stabilize, if not improve.

Most people find that their dog's annual checkup at the veterinarian is all that's needed, unless there's an injury or accident of some sort. Vet bills drop dramatically as you see those pesky disorders disappear; your dog's eyes, skin, and coat clear up, and his weight becomes stable — with all the attendant decreases in diseases due to excess weight. You can also save on expensive (and toxic) flea baths and dips, prescription foods, and medications as your dog becomes healthier.

Guardians feeding Paleo-type diets (raw meat, raw bones, and veggies) have specifically reported resolution of the following conditions, which previously made them "frequent fliers" at their veterinarian's office:

- Allergies
- Anxiety
- Apathy
- Coccidia, whipworms, and kennel cough in a shelter puppy
- Copper toxicosis
- Demodectic mange
- Dental disease
- Diarrhea
- Dry coat
- Ear infections
- Excessive shedding
- Fading coat color and reddening of black coat
- Gassiness (belching and flatulence)
- Greasy coat
- Hot spots (lick granulomas)
- Hyperactivity
- Inflammatory bowel disease (IBD)
- Itchy skin
- Lethargy

- Mental dullness
- Obesity
- Pododermatitis (inflammation of the feet; specifically, the skin between the toes)
- Scabs and rashes
- Seizures
- Skin infections (including staph)

Your vet may miss seeing you and your dog so often, but a good vet will be delighted that your dog is enjoying truly better health.

CHAPTER 4
THE PROBLEMS WITH COMMERCIAL DOG FOOD

To understand the importance of the Paleo Dog Diet as the most appropriate, natural, and healthful way to feed your dog, you have to understand how far short of the ideal that commercial pet food truly falls. In fact, there's good evidence that it's making our dogs sick and cutting their lives short.

Commercial dog food comes in many forms, and the vast majority are heavily processed, including canned, dry, semi-moist ("bits"), and the various combinations thereof. They're convenient, and many are relatively inexpensive to buy. (Their true cost is a very different matter.) Veterinarians recommend them, and they're incessantly advertised in the media, especially in magazines and on TV. Most people don't know the difference between one and another; they shop based on cost and marketing appeal. But if we're looking for the healthiest diet possible for our dogs, commercial food likely won't be in the running.

So, why is commercial pet food *not* a good choice for your dog?

REGULATION AND STANDARDS

The pet food industry is fond of saying it's the most highly regulated industry in the country, but that's nonsense. And the fact that it's not true actually has a huge impact on your dog. This is not a glamorous topic, but it's worth becoming educated about it. We'll try to make it as painless as possible.

The FDA has broad responsibility for all food, including animal feed and pet food. However, despite the Federal Food, Drug, and Cosmetic Act, requiring all food — for humans and animals — to be pure and unadulterated, the FDA has put "compliance policies" into place that allow a wide variety of heinous ingredients to be added to pet food, as long as they are processed to kill bacteria and other pathogenic organisms. For example, according to the Center for Veterinary Medicine (a division of the FDA): "The Center has permitted other aesthetic variables in dealing with animal feed, as for instance the use of properly treated *insect or rodent contaminated food* for animal feed [emphasis added]."[1]

Here's another one: "Some pet foods

91

contain the rendered (cooked) remains of diseased animals or animals that have died 'other than by slaughter.' "[2] This means animals that have died on the farm, or on the truck, or just outside the slaughterhouse door — no matter why they died, or how long they have been dead. This includes so-called "4-D meat" from animals that are dead, dying, disabled, or diseased.

So, we're not getting any help from the feds in regard to keeping pet foods clean and wholesome. Who else is out there?

Well, there's the Association of American Feed Control Officials (AAFCO). You've seen the statements on cans or bags of dog food: "Animal feeding tests using AAFCO procedures substantiate that [name of product] provides complete and balanced nutrition for [life stage]," or "[Name of product] is formulated to meet the nutritional levels established by the AAFCO Dog Food Nutrient Profiles for [life stage]."[3]

Many people assume that the AAFCO is the agency that polices the pet food industry, but it has no regulatory power whatsoever; it cannot test, approve, or ban foods. It is a nongovernmental, nonregulatory, voluntary organization of feed control officials (FCOs) from each state (as well as several other countries) and representatives of federal agencies such as the FDA.

The AAFCO exists to provide a forum for discussion by all interested parties about quality and standardization for animal feed and pet food. It also provides nutritional standards for pet foods, guidelines for feed and pet food manufacturing and labeling, and enforcement suggestions for the real regulators at the state level — the FCOs.

The AAFCO encourages experts from many different fields to advise the state FCOs. Formerly called "liaisons," these advisors come from the pet food industry, including the Washington, DC, lobbying group Pet Food Institute, as well as the grain and feed industries, the rendering industry, laboratories, farm co-ops, and other groups with an interest in the AAFCO's decisions.

The presence of so many folks who would like to influence the FCOs to benefit themselves worries many animal welfare activists. However, only the FCOs and the FDA and USDA representatives are *voting* members of the AAFCO. At AAFCO meetings, which are held twice a year, advisors often speak on issues when they have an interest or a stake in the outcome. Advisors' comments are considered by the FCOs, and then the issue is voted on by the FCOs, but they are not "pawns of industry." And they actually appreciate input from consumers.

Perhaps the AAFCO's biggest legacy to the FCOs as well as consumers has been the development of two tools for the standardization of pet food formulation. Most, but not all, states have adopted the AAFCO's model language, and require foods sold there to adhere to one of the two AAFCO standards. But remember, it is the state FCOs who check to see whether the food makers are compliant with the standards.

1. **Nutrient Profiles.** The first standard is the AAFCO Nutrient Profiles, which set the levels of 36 nutrients that must be present in formulated pet foods. Although the Nutrient Profile system has done a lot to standardize the business of pet food production, it's not without its critics. The Nutrient Profiles were officially updated as of January 1, 2014 (but they are based on data that is already a decade old).

2. **Feeding Tests.** The second method for pet food formulation addresses those concerns, but contains some loopholes as well. The AAFCO

developed a protocol for a 6-month feeding trial that can be used as a tool to determine whether a food can sustain life in a target test population — such as dogs or cats in all life stages, or specific stages of growth or maintenance. (The growth/lactation protocol is only 10 weeks; more extensive blood tests are required.) The test population is fed nothing but water and the test food for 6 months, and if the subjects test normal on weight and a few blood tests, the food passes. This method theoretically demonstrates that the food is palatable and digestible enough to maintain life in the test population — something the Nutrient Profiles do not require.

However, the feeding test requires only eight test subjects, and only six must finish the trial. Many nutritional deficiencies or overdoses would not appear in this short period; the feed's fitness for maintaining longevity and reproductive or multigenerational health would not be demonstrated. (In reality, most pet food companies using feeding tests use many more animals than the eight required, and the major manufacturers do conduct generational studies.)

The feeding test system has long been considered the gold standard, but it turned to fool's gold when the AAFCO passed the "family rule." Feeding tests are expensive and time consuming, and pet food companies don't really want to pay for them. But they know that consumers believe that foods with the feeding test statement on the label are more trusted by both consumers and veterinarians. The family rule allows any food that is nutritionally similar to a food that passed a feeding test to get the same label. In other words, there is no way for consumers to know whether a food bearing the label was actually tested or is only a very distant cousin to one that was tested.

Obviously, this system can miss a lot of potential problems. A food that meets the Nutrient Profiles may or may not pass a feeding trial; and foods that have passed a feeding trial don't have to meet the specifications of the Nutrient Profiles.[4] So for all the ballyhoo about pet food companies knowing everything there is to know about pet nutrition, the reality is that they don't.

In case you hadn't noticed, there is a whole lot of advertising hype going on about pet foods. And watching those ads, even on cable TV, isn't going to enlighten you!

"Meat is #1." Many dry foods advertise that they contain "meat" (such as chicken or beef) as the first or top ingredient. However, because of the high water content of fresh meat — not to mention the fact that it is further diluted during processing — the actual percentage of real meat is very, very small. It turns out that the first named *meal* is usually the primary protein source in dry foods, even though it may not be close to the top of the list.

"Human grade." A lot of pet foods claim that they contain human-grade ingredients. In practice, this claim has a federal standard that dog food does not meet, but since the FDA is not currently enforcing it, the pet food companies get away with using the term.

The USDA is the agency responsible for inspecting manufacturing plants making human food. However, as soon as the food is designated for animal consumption, that responsibility passes to the FDA. In reality, only one pet food company can legitimately use the term "human grade": the Honest

Kitchen, which can call its ingredients "human grade" because they are maintained in a human-edible condition from beginning to end.

Other companies may *start* with human-grade ingredients, but at some point (usually the minute they leave the slaughterhouse) they become "human inedible" or "pet food grade." The same applies to "USDA inspected" or similar phrases. The implication is that the food is made using ingredients that are passed by the USDA for human consumption, but there are many ways around this. For instance, a facility might be USDA-inspected during the day, but the pet food is made at night after the inspector is gone. When an ingredient leaves the human-food processing facility and the jurisdiction of the USDA, it is no longer human grade.

"Glam" ingredients. Many high-end foods contain ingredients like avocado, spinach, blueberries, cranberries, flaxseeds, parsley, and other items you might buy for yourself in the grocery store. The quality of these ingredients is not specified, and the levels are typically too small to add anything to the nutritional value of the food. Such ingredients are strictly window dressing; they're included only to make the food appealing to *you,* not for any health benefits to your dog. (Actually, that's the purpose behind *all* dog food advertising . . . and it will stay that way until our dogs learn how to use credit cards to buy their own food!)

Hidden sources. As we sadly learned from the 2007 pet food recalls, in the modern global economy, ingredients can be sourced from just about anywhere. China, Indonesia, and even Africa are now common sources of animal protein ingredients. Imported ingredients are almost never inspected, so poor quality, contaminated, and even adulterated (deliberately altered) ingredients can easily slip into U.S. manufacturing facilities. Or, food can be manufactured overseas and shipped straight into U.S. ports.

The trick is that regardless of the quality or source, the name of the ingredient on the label remains exactly the same. This is how manufacturers of cheap knockoffs and private-label brands try to fool you into thinking their food is as good as that expensive natural brand. And price isn't a good test either; some of the worst offenders cost the most!

Unfortunately, it's almost impossible to tell the wheat from the chaff when it comes to commercial dog food. The labels on many products are deliberately vague and intended to mislead. Fortunately, there is a better alternative, which we'll get to in Chapter 8!

INGREDIENTS

Over the years, research in canine nutrition has subtly shifted from figuring out a dog's minimum nutritional requirements to finding ways to satisfy them for the least cost. This is partly due to the free market culture of greed, and partly to law: The first and only mandated goal of a corporation is to make a profit for its shareholders. So when corporations tell you that their primary goal is to make dog food that will keep your dog healthy and happy, they are either lying or violating federal law. So much for truth in advertising!

Pet food has always been made from the leftovers of human food processing, but as the human food industry has become much better at squeezing every fragment of human-edible stuff from the raw materials, the nutritional value of those leftovers has drastically declined.

Early canned dog food was 100 percent meat (usually horse meat); vitamins and minerals weren't added until the need for them became apparent. Over the years, more and more meat was diverted into human food channels, meaning that less and less of it was available for our carnivorous canines. Research proved that puppies could get by on a diet containing just 15 percent protein.[5] Protein is the most expensive ingredient, and meat protein is the most expensive of all. Grain and vegetable proteins and meat by-products gradually replaced meat as a pet food ingredient. Today, cheap, mass-market dog foods may not contain any actual meat at all!

The quality of pet food ingredients is widely variable, but better-quality ingredients produce better results. For example, one study found that more of a poor-quality protein was needed to produce satisfactory results than less of a better-quality protein blend.[6] Duh! Today, the pet food industry knows exactly how to get away with using the cheapest ingredients without causing overt ill health in the dogs consuming those ingredients. And we accept our dogs' health as "normal" when, in truth, it is merely average — and average is a pretty poor standard indeed.

But how do you get a dog to eat a meatless brew of grain fractions and animal parts that, in the wild, would usually be left for scavengers? That's one thing pet food makers are extremely good at: making bad ingredients taste good!

Protein sounds like it should be a simple item, but it's not. All living organisms contain protein; it's just a matter of how much. Meat and eggs contain large amounts of highly digestible protein. Other animal parts, such as liver and intestines (aka by-products), also contain a lot of protein, although it's not quite as good in terms of quality or digestibility. Grains such as corn and wheat, and vegetables like peas and potatoes, contain small amounts of protein, but clever humans have figured out how to separate and concentrate those plant proteins for use in pet food. Yes, they'll meet your dog's minimum protein requirements, but they are a far cry from the animal sources of protein your dog needs for good health.[7]

The quality of animal-source proteins ranges from simply not wanted for human consumption to diseased and disgusting. Just as there are several USDA grades of meat (Prime, Choice, Select, and Standard), there are grades of meat meal, poultry meal, by-product meal, etc. They vary in quality and nutritional content, but most important to manufacturers, they vary greatly in price.

You may have read that "chicken meal" is a desirable ingredient in dog food, and

you'll find it in a wide range of pro
Chicken meal (a subset of poultry m
a rendered product that includes fle
skin, with or without bones. However, even
products that look decent, based on their
labels, may actually be bottom-of-the-barrel
in quality, particularly if the ingredients are
imported from China. Copackers and
manufacturers that make multiple brands
and private labels are well known for using
cheap ingredients, but even reputable
brands may be hiding poor-quality proteins
behind their labels. The fact is, there just
aren't enough truly high-quality protein
ingredients in existence to be used in the
thousands of foods claiming to contain
them.

Fats that end up in pet food come from
several sources, and are nearly all omega-6
fats. Animal fat is a product of rendering.
Some renderers are closely associated with
slaughterhouses and process only a few species, such as poultry or cattle; fats from such
facilities will have a name like "chicken fat"
or "beef tallow." Vegetable oils and used
restaurant grease also end up in pet food.[8]
Fat makes food taste good; dogs love it. But
Dr. Demien Dressler, a veterinarian known
as the "dog cancer vet," claims that the three
dietary factors leading to an increased risk

103

cancer are "excessive consumption of omega-6 polyunsaturated fatty acids (PUFAs), inefficient consumption of omega-3 PUFAs, and excessive calories in food."[9]

For many years, there have been persistent rumors that dead dogs and cats from shelters and veterinary clinics are rendered and put into pet food. The FDA admits that this is permissible, but not "condoned." To try to assuage the rumors, the FDA did extensive testing and found no evidence of dog or cat DNA in pet food. However, in 2013, this very scenario was found to be occurring in Spain. But seriously, folks, given all the other garbage that ends up in pet food, nothing is impossible!

Currently, the American human diet typically has a ratio of omega-6s to omega-3s of between 20:1 and 30:1. But the natural or optimal ratio is less than 5:1. Since pet food derives from human food waste, it also tends to be heavy in omega-6s, with little or no omega-3s. Some manufacturers add fish meal or other sources of omega-3s, but not enough to achieve a proper balance. This highly disproportionate fat ratio leads to

inflammation, which provides an i̇
environment for the development of canċ
and other chronic diseases.[10]

Carbohydrates are abundant in commercial pet food, even though adult dogs have no requirement for carbs at all. Grains and/or starchy vegetables in dry food have two purposes: first, to get the right consistency of dough for the extruder (the machine that makes kibble); and second, to provide a cheap source of calories (or "energy," as the nutritionists prefer to call it). But excessive simple carbohydrates are to blame for most of the weight problems we see in pets.

The other big problem with carbohydrates is that cancer loves them; research suggests that most, if not all, cancers have a sweet tooth, lymphoma in particular.[11] All carbohydrates (except fiber) eventually break down into sugar — specifically glucose, which the body uses for energy. Cancer also uses carbs for energy. However, dogs can also use fat and protein for energy, while cancer cannot. So it makes sense to restrict carbohydrates, not only to starve out cancer that already exists but also to prevent it from developing in the first place.[12]

The natural Paleo Dog Diet contains less than 10 percent carbohydrates, while most dry dog foods have 30 to 50 percent, and even most canned dog foods contain way more carbs than are good for dogs (or cats or people).[13]

ADDITIVES

There are 27 classes of additives that may be used in pet food, including anticaking agents, antioxidants, color additives, drying agents, emulsifiers, flavor enhancers, palatants, pelleting agents and binders, petroleum derivatives, pH control agents, preservatives, stabilizers, texturizers, and thickeners.[14] Dog foods must appeal first to the humans who buy and prepare them.

Looking at preservatives, we find the first and greatest divide among dry dog foods: those that use chemical preservatives and those that use natural ones instead. The goal of all is to create a product with a shelf life of 12 to 18 months, and for this, chemicals do a better job. Common synthetic preservatives include:

- BHA (butylated hydroxytoluene) and BHT (butylated hydroxyanisol), petroleum derivatives that accumulate in body tissue and may cause liver enlargement and reduced DNA synthesis and increase the risk of cancer. On the plus side, their antioxidant properties may actually reduce the incidence of cancer in some cases. BHA is considered more toxic than BHT, but BHT can cross the blood-brain barrier, and it interferes with blood clotting. They may trigger hypersensitivity (allergies) and may have carcinogenic properties.

- Ethoxyquin, a controversial ingredient in pet foods. It was originally used as an herbicide and in rubber manufacturing. Ethoxyquin has been causing a stir for decades, and most pet food manufacturers have replaced it with natural preservatives (vitamins C and E) in their products, but some "veterinarian prescribed" diets still use it.
- Propylene glycol, a solvent and "humectant," a water-holding ingredient used to preserve soft "bits" as well as dry dog food. It's a topical irritant in humans, and so toxic to cats that it's banned in cat food. It's most famously used as antifreeze.

CONTAMINANTS

A major pet food concern is the potential presence of toxic and illness-causing substances and organisms.

Drugs administered to livestock, the pentobarbital used to kill shelter dogs and cats (as well as some horses and livestock), pesticides and fertilizers on grains, molds, heavy metals, and other toxins are not prohibited in pet foods — not regulated, not checked for, and in many cases, not affected or inactivated by processing. While there are no documented cases of clinical disease or harm to animals eating these foods, clearly there are grounds for concern over these contaminants, especially the potential for adverse effects from daily, low-level consumption over many years. The increase over time of chronic diseases such as cancer in dogs and cats may have a nutritional component that has not yet been recognized by the veterinary community.

Chemical residues are allowed without limit in pet foods. This means that grains and other crops that are condemned for human consumption because of excess residues of fertilizers, pesticides, or other agricultural chemicals can be and are used in animal feeds, including pet food.

Toxic chemicals, including polybrominated diphenyl ethers (fire retardants), organochlorines, phthalates, and perfluorochemicals (Teflon), have been found in pets. Not in pet food — in *pets*! These chemicals may have toxic effects at far lower levels than previously considered safe. The Environmental Working Group conducted a study of pets and found that dogs' blood and urine samples were contaminated with "35 chemicals . . . including 11 carcinogens, 31 chemicals toxic to the reproductive system, and 24 neurotoxins. The carcinogens are of particular concern, since dogs have much higher rates of many kinds of cancer than do people, including 35 times more skin cancer, 4 times more breast tumors, 8 times more bone cancer, and twice the incidence of leukemia, according to the Texas A&M Veterinary Medical Center."[15] Some of these pollutants enter pets through air and water, but many are directly consumed in pet food, such as fire retardants, which are found at high levels in some fish and poultry by-products.

BPA (bisphenol A) is a toxic compound found in an assortment of plastics, including the plastic that lines many human and pet food cans. Some manufacturers have removed BPA from pet food cans, but in many cases they have simply substituted similar (and equally, if not more, toxic) compounds.

Antibiotics and other drugs are commonly fed to livestock. According to numerous estimates, approximately 80 percent of all antibiotic use in the United States is for livestock.[16] Most of the 40-plus FDA-approved antibiotics are given for nontherapeutic purposes:

- To promote growth or other desired characteristics
- To compensate for the increased disease potential in factory-animals crowded together in unsanitary conditions

Widespread subtherapeutic use of antibiotics has contributed to the rapid rise of resistant bacteria, making treatment of food-borne illness in people a challenge. These drugs are directly entering the human food chain when people eat meat from those animals, and of course, our dogs are eating them, too.

Nevertheless, after numerous petitions over 34 years asking the FDA to limit antibiotic use in food-producing animals, in 2012 the agency decided to deny all of them, saying that it would cost too much to withdraw approvals for an array of antibiotics used as growth promoters and disease "preventatives" that are fed to billions of poultry and livestock for the sole purpose of increasing profit. Such subclinical antibiotic use contributes to the development of antibiotic-resistant bacteria such as MRSA (methicillin-resistant *Staphylococcus aureus*), not to mention the threat it poses to humans who are allergic to penicillin and other drugs being used in food animals. Fortunately, a federal court slapped the FDA upside the head and ordered it to do its job!

Worse still, drugs such as penicillin and pentobarbital, the drug used for euthanasia, pass through pet food processing unchanged. The FDA studied pentobarbital and found an association between a positive test for pentobarbital and the presence of particular ingredients, particularly animal fat, meat meal, and bone meal.[17]

Bacteria. Outright contamination of food by bacteria and their associated endotoxins is another serious concern. High-temperature processing kills most bacteria, but it does not affect bacterial endotoxins, fungal mycotoxins, or *Clostridia* spores.

In just the past few years, there have been dozens of recalls of dry dog food because of *Salmonella* contamination. Dry food is essentially sterile when it exits the extruder, but unless scrupulous hygiene and air quality controls are in place, it's easy for the food to be recontaminated.

Genetically modified organisms (GMOs) are widespread in the United States, Canada, and Asia. In the United States, GMO products are unlabeled and, for all practical purposes, unregulated. There are valid concerns about the serious reduction in the biodiversity of crops, which may make our entire agricultural system susceptible to new pathogens. This in turn could lead to widespread crop failures and financial disaster for our economy. And that's before we even think about the potential health consequences!

As of 2012, 94 percent of soybeans and 88 percent of corn planted in the United States is GMO. Most of it goes into livestock feed, which ends up in both human and pet food. Of course, leftover and out-of-date food may be recycled into either animal feed or pet food. Your dog may be getting a double whammy of GMOs: the corn-fed meat, by-products, and dairy products in his food, on top of the GMO corn and soy used directly as a major dog food ingredient. A recent study clearly showed serious toxicity in rats fed GMO corn.[18]

As bad as you might think GMOs are, they're way worse. Contrary to claims, the FDA never adequately studied GMOs, and it is still operating under old policies put in place when the new technology promised increased yields, lower costs, and less pesticide use. None of these promises has come true, and in fact, quite the opposite has occurred. We're now using more pesticides than ever, because super-weeds and super-pests have developed resistance and now require more and stronger chemicals to suppress them. There are many other problems as well, including documented organ damage and tumor growth in animal studies. The *Bt (Bacillus thuringiensis)* pesticide that we were assured would affect only targeted insect pests also harms nontarget species like bees and butterflies and causes damage to animal and human cells.[19]

According to the Grocery Manufacturers Association, GMOs are now present in 75 to 80 percent of U.S conventional processed food — from breakfast cereal to frozen dinners. If the label doesn't say "organic" or "GMO-free," it is almost certain to be contaminated. (There is even GMO fresh produce, but so far it's limited to Hawaiian and Chinese papaya, and some varieties of zucchini, yellow squash, and corn on the cob.)

Irradiation is an FDA-approved method of reducing bacterial contamination in the food supply. Contamination, particularly by

Salmonella, is a serious problem that has only increased under the federal Hazard Analysis and Critical Control Point guidelines that have governed food processing in the United States since 1995. Meat and meat by-products destined for animal feed and pet food may also be irradiated. The FDA promulgated a specific rule in April 2001 allowing irradiation of pet foods. While the World Health Organization and the U.S. government have gone to great lengths to convince consumers that irradiated food is perfectly safe, a significant body of scientific evidence shows that it is not. Australia recently rescinded its rule requiring irradiation of all imported pet food after 90 cats became ill from eating irradiated food; it was the third such incident since 1998.[20] Ionizing radiation destroys nutrients, increases carcinogens, and creates harmful free radicals. While irradiation is touted as a solution for bacterial contamination in the meatpacking industry, the truth is that it is being used *instead* of adequate sanitation and hygienic procedures.[21]

Mold toxins, such as aflatoxin, have caused many recalls over the years, and are still going on today. Hundreds of dogs have died as a result of aflatoxin poisoning since the 1990s. Yet, the pet food industry as a whole

114

has not bothered to improve its testing, despite giving consumers numerous assurances and promises to the contrary. *Food Safety News,* commenting on just one of many widespread recalls, stated, "All the companies have said that, to date, no illnesses or adverse effects have been reported in connection with the recalled dog food, but did not explain why dog food was on the market for more than a year before it was tested for aflatoxins."[22]

Industrial and other toxic wastes containing heavy metals such as arsenic, mercury, cadmium, lead and other heavy metals, dioxins, and even radioactive materials have been "recycled" as fertilizer for years, all perfectly legally. The crops so fertilized may be used for livestock feed, as well as for direct human consumption. This certainly has serious implications for human health as well as for our dogs.

Another material used in feed for livestock is, somewhat shockingly, animal wastes. Fecal matter contains undigested plant material as well as large quantities of dead bacteria — which are considered to be an edible protein source. Poultry, swine, and ruminant waste and litter, containing up to 30 percent dirt, rocks, and wood shavings, are all considered acceptable ingredients for animal feeds. In fact, animal feed is allowed to contain up to 40 percent straw, wood shavings, and other bedding materials as "sources of fiber." The urine soaking these materials is a "non-protein nitrogen" that is an acceptable substitute for actual protein.[23] Bear in mind that the animals eating these materials are going into the human food chain; the leftovers go to pet food.

The declining nutritional quality of crops is, or should be, a huge concern for us all. Even if cropland is not contaminated by toxin-containing fertilizers, the current non-sustainable agricultural practice of heavy artificial fertilizer and chemical pesticide use is deteriorating the quality and nutritional value of the food supply — not just for pets but for humans as well. Much of our farmland has essentially been chemically sterilized, stripped of its symbiotic bacteria, fungi, and other organic matter, and then saturated with just enough synthetic fertilizers to sustain plant life. Crop plants may look good, but the nutrient content and value of produce has decreased dramatically over the past few decades. Moreover, our lands and waters are heavily contaminated by runoff from chemical-saturated fields, as well as by animal waste products that come from intensive confinement and factory-farming operations around the country. These contaminants are sprayed back onto croplands in the irrigation water, where they can be taken up by plants. From there, they climb back up the food chain: into livestock feed, which the animals convert into the meat on our tables and the food in our dogs' food bowls.

Acrylamide is a toxic compound formed at cooking temperatures of about 250°F in foods containing certain sugars and the amino acid asparagine (found in large amounts in potatoes and cereal grains), mainly because of the Maillard (browning) reaction. Acrylamide causes cancer in laboratory animals and is considered a potential human carcinogen. Most dry pet foods contain up to 50 percent or more cereal grain ingredients, and they are processed at high temperatures (over 200°F during rendering and again at high pressure during extrusion; baked foods are cooked at well over 500°F); these are perfect conditions for the Maillard reaction. In fact, the Maillard reaction is sometimes considered desirable in the production of pet food because it imparts a particular taste that is especially palatable to pets. The content and potential effects of acrylamide in pet foods are as yet unknown. It may not surprise you to discover that nobody is trying very hard to find out, either.

Foreign ingredients are just one more thing to worry about — and it's a big thing. In 2007, we learned, to our great sorrow, that other countries don't do things the same way we do. Wheat gluten from China, deliberately spiked with melamine to fake a higher protein content, sickened and killed tens of thousands of dogs and cats. Nevertheless, massive quantities of pet food ingredients are still imported from China and other countries. In fact, such imports rose by 29 percent between 2010 and 2011. In just one month (February 2011), U.S. companies imported nearly $22 million in pet food and treat ingredients from China (which supplies 70 percent of all such imports). An article in *PetFood Industry* magazine claims that "pet owners and manufacturers realize the necessity of such products."[24] Excuse us? No, we don't! We understand the necessity for makers of cheap pet food to use cheap ingredients, but reasonable people have an expectation that when they seek out and pay good money for supposedly high-quality products, those products are not from China!

Country-of-origin information, while required on human food, is not to be found

118

on pet food labels. Even foods that claim to be locally sourced may be using ingredients that are themselves from other countries. For example, some amino acids simply aren't made in the United States and must be imported from Asia. Virtually all vitamin premixes used in the pet food industry contain imported ingredients.

Importing cheaper versions of standard ingredients is a major way that pet food companies save money. Yet there is no way to tell from the label whether inexpensive foreign ingredients have been used, and many companies will fudge the truth when asked directly, saying "we source our ingredients from the United States," without mentioning that their *suppliers* may not.

TREATS

Studies show that 99 percent of dogs are given treats, and there's nothing wrong with that. But there are things you can do to moderate the number of treat calories your dog is getting without making your pet (or you!) feel deprived.

1. Treats should never amount to more than 10 percent of your dog's daily caloric intake.
2. Break larger treats into smaller

pieces. Your pet will quickly adjust to the new size, and feel just as pampered.

3. Give a lower-calorie treat, or try treats made from dehydrated chicken, liver, or other meats that add primarily protein and little or no carbs.

4. Restrict rawhide, marrow bones, and other animal parts. Many of them are very high in fat and carry a huge load of calories.

5. Avoid all treats made in China and all "jerky" type treats. Hundreds of dogs have died from an unknown contaminant in chicken jerky made in China. The FDA has been issuing warnings since 2007. A few products were recalled but put back on shelves without alteration. At the time of this writing, it is thought that antibiotic residues in the Chinese chicken are to blame. These antibiotics are legal in China but illegal in the United States.

To your dog, it's really more about the attention and love from you that are associated with treats than about the treat itself. Pats and hugs are calorie free, so no limits!

What about Rawhides, Bully Sticks, and Chews?

We've all seen them at the local market and pet store, and sometimes at the vet clinic as well, but they come with controversy. You may have heard the warnings and been told to always supervise your dog when he chews such products, as they can break apart into sharp pieces or otherwise cause a blockage. You know them by names such as rawhide chews, Greenies, Nylabone, cow hooves, pig ears, and many others. They come in all sizes and shapes for your size, breed, and age of dog. Many people opt for one of these chews because they have been frightened away from the healthy choice of raw meat and raw bones, having never been told that it is the cooked bones that cause the problems, for the most part because they splinter. Let's take a look at these chew toys.

Rawhide chews are the skin of the cow with the hair removed. Depending on what country the rawhide comes from, the skin can be contaminated with feces, bacteria, pesticides, and heavy metals that may adversely affect your dog. To prepare the rawhide, it is soaked in a caustic lime solution, followed by bleach. It may or may not have artificial smoke flavor and color added. A chunk of rawhide can cause choking; if swallowed, it can scrape and irritate the dog's throat and or esophagus.

Greenies, the toothbrush-shaped dog treats, have become popular thanks to masterful marketing, but they won't clean your dog's teeth. Inappropriately sized Greenies can lodge in your dog's esophagus. There is nothing Paleo about them; they're full of fractionated proteins, "hydrogenated starch hydrogenate," feel-good "glamour" ingredients like cranberry fiber, and synthetic vitamins.

Nylabones are hard, plasticlike products, which have been reported to break or become lodged in the back of a dog's throat, potentially causing a severe obstruction. The Nylabones that are clear are reported to be impossible to be seen on radiographs (x-rays). It is possible that an attending veterinarian cannot see the blockage without resorting to exploratory surgery. Because they have a very hard consistency, they can also damage your dog's teeth.

Animal parts that would otherwise be discarded (or turned into meat-and-bone meal) have been turned into a lucrative side business of slaughter as dog chews or treats. Such parts include bullies or pizzles (made from dried penises, usually from cattle), pig ears, hooves, skin, hide, or jerky. These products are not cooked to a temperature that kills bacteria, so contamination, particularly with *Salmonella,* is common. Your dog may not display symptoms, but you can get sick from handling them. Like other chew-type treats, they pose a choking hazard for your dog. Furthermore, they often have a strong odor that you may not enjoy, and they can stain your dog's paws as well as your carpet and furniture.

CHAPTER 5
MENACES OF MODERN LIFE

One thing's for sure: There are a lot of things in modern life that the original Paleo Dogs didn't have to — and weren't built to — cope with. The chemicals used on our yards and in household products, air pollution, and radiation are just a few of them. In addition, modern veterinary care can be pretty poisonous. Paleo Dogs never had to deal with flea treatments, heartworm preventives, anesthetics, or surgery.

Let's take a look at some of these factors in more detail.

HOME AND YARD TOXINS

Many of the products we take for granted are actually toxic, such as household cleansers, disinfectants, and polishers, and lawn and garden pesticides and fertilizers. Many of them are mislabeled or lack adequate warnings. Over time, exposure to toxic chemicals can contribute to the development of cancer, birth defects, genetic changes, allergies, and many other disorders, to say nothing of a generally weakened immune system.

Because of their size and physiology, children and pets are the most vulnerable to chemical toxicity. Smaller size means a higher rate of metabolism. Many pollutants are heavier than air and are therefore found in greater concentration lower to the ground, where children and animals are apt to receive much higher exposure.

Cleaning products are among the most hazardous materials found in the home. Consider replacing household chemicals with nontoxic, biodegradable substitutes. Check your local health food store for safe products, or make your own from safe ingredients.

Teflon is another household hazard. It exudes toxic fumes when it overheats — enough to kill pet birds, and certainly not good for you or your dog! Use cast iron, ceramic, glass, or stainless steel (but not aluminum) for cooking.

Obviously, smoke from cigarettes, cigars, pipes, and other smoking materials are highly toxic to both you and your dog. All smoking must be done outside and well away from doors and windows so that

Toxic Product	Safe Product	Comment
Air fresheners	Aromatherapy hydrosols	Air fresheners, potpourri, scented candles, essential oil diffusers, and incense may be offensive to your dog's highly sensitive nose
Cleansers	Lemon juice	Cuts grease
	Vinegar (white distilled)	Grease-cutting cleanser for floors and hard surfaces; glass cleaner
	Borax	Non-scratching scouring cleanser
Deodorizers	Baking soda	Deodorizer
Disinfectants	Bleach (diluted 1:32, or 4 ounces in 1 gallon of water)	The top disinfectant; kills bacteria and viruses; once dry, it is totally safe
	Vinegar (white distilled)	Kills bacteria, algae, viruses, and mold
Fabric softener	Vinegar (white distilled)	Natural fabric softener
Insect repellent	Neem tree oil	Antibacterial insect repellent
Polish	Borax	Deodorizer; mold inhibitor; rust stain remover
	Beeswax	Polish for floors and furniture
	Jojoba oil	Furniture polish
	Toothpaste (not gel)	Silver and other metal polish

smoke doesn't drift back into the house. And, seriously . . . if you won't quit for your own or your family's sake, please quit for your dog's!

Marijuana is also toxic to dogs, who lack the liver pathways to metabolize it. Pot doesn't make them high — it just makes them sick. And the smoke is just plain irritating to their sensitive noses. Always make sure that all drugs (legal or otherwise!) are securely stored out of reach of pets and children. *Note:* Trash cans are definitely *not* secure. Veterinarians are investigating certain strains of pot for pain relief in pets, but this is currently not a legitimate use.[1]

A virtually unrecognized source of potential irritation and possible poison to your dog is the common air freshener. Such products are really just chemical soups designed to fool your sense of smell. And while a hint of lavender may be relaxing to humans, there's no guarantee that it will have a similar effect on animals. Some odors that humans find agreeable may be aversive to pets; and the reverse is also true (just think for a moment about the things your dog loves to sniff the most — other dogs' behinds and all varieties of waste come immediately to mind).

A dog's sense of smell is at least 40 times

more perceptive than ours. To a sensitive nose, artificial and even many natural scents, such as diffused essential oils, must feel like living with the stereo turned up full blast day and night. The problem is compounded when multiple scent products are used throughout the house, leaving nowhere for the dog to go to get away from them. So, while occasionally burning a scented candle or stick of incense won't hurt, please avoid air fresheners.

According to research, companion animals' levels of toxic metals and other contaminants have reached dangerous proportions.[2] You may wish to have a heavy metal or mineral analysis — by atomic absorption rather than flame photometry, which is not as accurate — done on a sample of your dog's fur. In any case, it's definitely worthwhile to detoxify your home for the benefit of all residents, whether two-legged or four!

VETERINARY MEDICINE

Veterinarians mean well. They will do their best to help your dog in case of illness or injury. And they do save lives and alleviate pain and suffering. The original Paleo Dogs never had that kind of care — and many of them died prematurely because of that lack. And Paleo Dogs didn't face the kind of challenges our modern dogs must cope with every day.

We certainly don't recommend never taking your dog to the vet; it would be extremely foolish to repudiate *all* the benefits of modern life! New problems need new therapies. But even the most well-intentioned or necessary treatment can have unwanted adverse effects. We recommend an educated, balanced approach to your dog's health. A little skepticism when it comes to some common veterinary treatments is definitely warranted. We do recommend developing a working relationship with a holistic veterinarian. Many will work with you over the phone. But you'll also need to find a good local vet to call on for routine care or in case of emergency — preferably one who is willing to work with you on the Paleo Dog Diet and Lifestyle.

Antibiotics. The misuse and overuse of antibiotics is a huge problem that is thought to cause or contribute to the rising number of antibiotic-resistant organisms and infections. An estimated 80 percent of antibiotics in the United States are given to livestock that will eventually end up in the human and pet food supply. That's bad enough! But individual veterinarians are also to blame when they prescribe antibiotics for

129

viral infections and other situations where they are clearly not indicated. The usual excuse is that "we're preventing secondary infections" — which are rare in adult dogs. However, young puppies with certain viral infections may be more vulnerable to secondary infection with bacteria and could potentially benefit from judicious use of antibiotics.

Antibiotics have recently been shown to actually aid the growth of harmful bacteria, such as *Salmonella* and *Clostridia* — two organisms that our dogs are commonly exposed to — in the gut. We always knew that when an animal takes an oral antibiotic, the drug kills off a large number of the normal, helpful bacteria in the gut. But new research finds that antibiotics create an environment that favors the bad bugs over the good ones, allowing the pathogenic bacteria to thrive. It doesn't matter if the antibiotic is given for an infected ear or toe: Its negative effects are still felt in the gut. The normal bacteria that are so important to health may never completely recover.[3]

If your dog does need antibiotics, you *must* simultaneously supplement with probiotics ("friendly" bacteria that normally live in the gut). The word *antibiotic* literally means "against life" — and they don't discriminate. These drugs kill all susceptible bacteria: the good, the bad, and the ugly! Repopulating the friendly gut bacteria helps to minimize the side effects of the drugs and to prevent diarrhea and other tummy problems. Give probiotics along with antibiotics (2 hours apart if possible; and preferably give the probiotics with food). Continue the probiotics for at least 2 weeks after the antibiotics are stopped (see Appendix A on page 419 and Resources on page 511).

Steroids. No, not the kind that athletes secretly use! The corticosteroids used in veterinary medicine are powerful anti-inflammatories. The most commonly used steroids include cortisone, prednisone, prednisolone, dexamethasone, and triamcinolone.

Normal side effects of steroids include increased appetite (which often results in weight gain), increased thirst, increased urination, and increased panting. These are also signs of Cushing's disease — a disorder in which the adrenal glands make too much of the body's own native steroid, cortisol. Iatrogenic Cushing's is the name for the disease when caused by excessive steroid use. Overuse may also cause high blood pressure, impaired wound healing, muscle weakness, thinning of skin, immune suppression (increased risk of infection), stomach ulcers, heart disease, hypertension, and psychological and/or behavior changes.

Nevertheless, as teachers in veterinary school say, "Better pred than dead." There are cases where steroid use is completely justified, such as to treat natural Addison's disease or an autoimmune condition where immediate suppression of the immune system is necessary.

There may be safer alternatives for many of the problems steroids are commonly used to treat, so please consult a holistic veterinarian if steroids have been recommended for your dog.

Pain medications. In contrast to the many overused drugs, pain medications are probably underutilized. Pain in animals has gone unrecognized and unacknowledged for most of history, and it is still not sufficiently treated by many veterinarians today, particularly those who graduated before the 1990s. A veterinary association focused on pain management wasn't even founded until 2003, didn't award its first certification until 2009, and still has fewer than 50 members — out of some 90,000 practicing American vets.[4] A survey published in 2000 found that less than half of veterinarians provided *any* postoperative pain management for canine spays or neuters.[5] By any standard, that is completely unacceptable.

Alternative medicine is particularly good at treating pain, and many therapies are consistent with the Paleo Dog Lifestyle. The earliest Paleo Dogs would have had access to herbs and nutraceuticals; they would also consume glucosamine and other joint-supporting nutrients as they chewed on the carcasses of their kills. And no doubt their early human companions would have used hands-on healing and energy therapies on their sick or injured companions — even if that's not what they called it. Contact your holistic vet to tailor a program for your dog.

DENTAL CARE

Even for Paleo Dogs who are eating the right diet and appropriate bones, dental care is still necessary. However, if your dog — like so many — is starting out with preexisting dental disease, both home and veterinary oral care will be needed. Proper dental care throughout every dog's life is essential to optimal health.

Dental disease is the most common health problem seen by veterinarians. By age 3, virtually all dogs have some degree of dental disease, ranging from a mild accumulation of tartar to severe infection and tooth loss.

Most pets would benefit from an annual dental exam and cleaning, but it is also important for you to take care of your pet's teeth at home.

Within hours after cleaning, bacteria start to recolonize the surface of the teeth. They secrete substances to attach themselves more firmly, and to protect themselves from the immune system. The combination of bacteria and their secretions is called plaque. If plaque is not removed, minerals in the saliva turn it into calculus (more commonly called tartar) within just 48 hours.

Some of the substances secreted by the bacteria cause inflammation of the gums (gingiva), resulting in gingivitis. If this is not treated, inflammation will progress and start to break down tissues in the mouth, leading to periodontal disease. Eventually, infection and erosion cause the teeth to decay, abscess, or fracture. All of these processes are painful to the animal.

While diet does play a role in dental disease, there is also a very strong genetic component. Small breeds, especially those with brachiocephalic (short-nosed) faces, often have overcrowded, decay-prone teeth. Some pets may need very little dental care, while others might require full cleanings under anesthesia once or even twice a year.

Excellent dental health requires help from your veterinarian as well as a commitment to home care from you. If your pet already has dental disease, the first step is to have his teeth cleaned under anesthesia by your veterinarian. While no surgery is risk free, modern anesthetics, together with appropriate monitoring and supportive care, make this a very low-risk procedure, even for older animals (who usually need it the most!).

The most reliable method of removing plaque and preventing dental disease at home is brushing the teeth. Ideally, you should do this daily. Brushing removes plaque on the outside of the crown (the above-gum portion) of the tooth and stimulates the gums to keep them healthy. However, plaque can still accumulate below the gumline, so an annual checkup and cleaning, if necessary, is still an essential part of your pet's dental health. Even if you don't see any problems, it is best to have your pet's teeth x-rayed and professionally cleaned prior to beginning a home care program, to make sure there are no painful areas in the mouth that might jeopardize your success.

Your veterinarian can show you how to

brush your dog's teeth, but it may still turn into a battle at home, which is the last thing you want! Here are a few tips to get you going:

- Buy a finger brush and toothpaste designed for pets. Do not use a human brush or even a pet brush on a stick; these can severely injure the gums without your knowing it (other than by your dog's very negative reaction!). Never use human toothpaste; the additives may be harmful to your dog, and the strong scent is likely to be objectionable.
- Since many dogs enjoy having their faces rubbed, gently stroking around the lips and corners of the mouth is a good place to start. (If your dog is shy about having this area touched, try Tellington T-Touch; see Resources on page 523.)
- Gradually extend your rubbing by slipping your finger under the lips and massaging the gums gently. Take this step slowly and back off immediately if your dog objects. You don't want to make this an unpleasant experience, so let your dog dictate how fast you progress.

- Put a little pet toothpaste on your finger as you rub. Most dogs love the taste.
- Put the brush on your finger with a little pet toothpaste. This will feel only slightly different from what you've been doing, and should be well tolerated. If not, remove the brush and go back a step. A piece of damp gauze can be substituted for the toothbrush.

It's best to brush every day; then if you miss a day, it's not a crisis. However, if you plan to brush every other day and *then* miss a session, you've lost several days that cannot be reclaimed, and plaque will have a good head start.

For some dogs, anesthesia-free teeth cleaning may be appropriate. Done correctly, it removes even subgingival plaque. However, changes in the bone, tooth roots, or periodontal tissues will not be detected.

Many dental care products are marketed for pets. Oral rinses, gels, and water additives will not control plaque by themselves. Treats do not contribute to dental health, even if they are labeled "tartar control." No proof of effectiveness is needed to put such a label on a treat; it's just a marketing gimmick.

Most dog chews — including nylon, rubber, and rawhide bones; and hooves — do little to reduce plaque accumulation, do nothing about plaque under the gumline, and can actually cause a dog's teeth to fracture. Broken teeth are a source of infection and pain to the dog, and an expense to you when they have to be extracted. If a dog swallows a chunk of any of these chews, it can cause a life-threatening intestinal blockage. If you have a ball-obsessed dog, don't let her chew on tennis balls; the fuzz rapidly wears teeth down.

Raw bones, given at appropriate intervals, can do an excellent job of removing and preventing tartar accumulation on exposed tooth surfaces. However, most dental disease starts under the gumline. Only an exam and x-rays under anesthesia will detect these hidden problems. See "Calcium and Raw Bones" on page 201 for more information on feeding bones.

Many serious health risks are associated with tooth decay. Bacteria living in these "slums" can enter the bloodstream and seed infection in critical organs like the heart, liver, and kidneys. Decayed and abscessed teeth are very painful and may hinder the animal from taking in enough nourishment, not to mention deteriorate the pet's quality of life. Many a cranky old dog has become happy and playful again after hidden dental problems were corrected.

Proper dental care is truly necessary to maintain optimal health and well-being.

MICROCHIPPING

Quite a lot of controversy surrounds the dangers of microchips, including their potential to cause cancer. This is mostly a risk in cats, but there have been quite a few reports of similar tumors in dogs.

There are several things you need to know to assess any information you may come upon.

1. The strains of mice used in studies showing tumor formation related to microchipping are bred to be especially susceptible to tumor formation. The fact that these particular mice develop tumors is not necessarily applicable to dogs.
2. Any injection, bruise, or other trauma has the potential to cause cancer (fibrosarcoma), even though the risk is very slight.
3. The chances of a dog getting loose or lost are much higher than the chances of a tumor resulting from a

microchip. Having a microchip (and hopefully additional identification like a collar) makes it much more likely you will be reunited with your pet.

4. Literally millions of dogs, cats, and horses have been microchipped in the past 2 decades. The majority of veterinarians do not see it as a problem.

5. To ensure the best result with minimal risk, the chip should be placed slightly off the midline and away from all acupuncture meridians, and an oral dose of homeopathic Ledum 30C should be given immediately afterward.

Many pets have been found years later and hundreds of miles away and, thanks to a tiny microchip, have been reunited with their families. Microchipping is "cheap insurance," and a good way to manage one of life's most awful risks — the loss of one's dog.

SPAYING AND NEUTERING

We'll be the first to say that spaying and neutering are necessary for dogs because of the terrible overpopulation problem; way too many healthy, loving dogs are killed every day in shelters. But in truth, that's a human problem: Irresponsible people are the issue, and dogs are the innocent victims.

Spaying and neutering have documented negative health implications that you must consider when deciding when — and if — you will have your dog surgically sterilized.[6] (Nonsurgical sterilization is on the horizon, so ask your veterinarian for options.)

First, of course, there are benefits. Your dog will not be able to reproduce (in terms of pet overpopulation, that's a good thing) and will be much less likely to develop cancers, infections, or other diseases of the reproductive organs, such as benign prostatic hypertrophy or pyometra (a life-threatening uterine infection). Spaying before the dog's first estrus (heat cycle) reduces the chance of mammary cancer, and if done before 2 1/2 years of age is still beneficial.

On the flip side, problems associated with spay/neuter (partly because of the loss of sex hormones) may include the following:

- Increased risk of several cancers, including osteosarcoma (bone cancer), hemangiosarcoma (a cancer of the

Caution: If any humans in the home are using medicated creams or gels, particularly those containing estrogen, progesterone, testosterone, or bio-identical hormones, be very careful around your pets (and children, too). Your dog's skin will absorb them just as well as yours does, and he may develop symptoms of an overdose if exposed. So be sure to cover these areas for at least 2 hours, and wash your hands thoroughly after application.

blood vessels), prostate cancer, and urinary tract tumors
- Increased risk of orthopedic disorders
- Obesity (removal of reproductive organs causes an instant drop in a dog's energy requirements because of the sudden cessation of hormone secretion; unless food intake is reduced postoperatively, chances of weight gain are high)
- Urinary tract infections
- Urinary incontinence (in spayed females)
- Increased risk or severity of age-related cognitive impairment

- Increased risk of hypothyroidism (although this is more likely because most dogs are also vaccinated at the time of surgery; vaccines are strongly implicated in the development of the disease)

Spayed and neutered dogs will also grow a little taller because of the delayed stoppage of bone growth, but whether that's a risk or a benefit is in the eye of the beholder. There is some evidence that sterilizing dogs before 5 1/2 months of age may be associated with a higher risk of hip dysplasia.

Of course, there are always risks with any surgery, such as bleeding and other complications. The anesthetics used today are far safer than those used in the past; anesthetic deaths are rare, but they do occur.

PARASITE PREVENTION AND TREATMENT

It's likely that ancient Paleo Dogs were troubled by parasites (using this term in its broadest sense, including fleas and other insects, ticks, worms, flukes, mites, protozoa, bacteria, viruses, and fungi) to some degree. Parasites are, after all, a natural part of the environment. In fact, new research suggests that some parasites may be beneficial and even necessary for optimal health.[7] The immune system normally keeps both internal and external parasites in check, while the parasites return the favor by keeping immunity strong and active. Parasites also help cull out the sick and weak animals — both predator and prey — to maintain a healthy population.

Even today, wolf populations are prevented from becoming too large through two main natural controls: food availability and parasites (not counting the current primary cause of wolf mortality — humans).[8] Overcrowding leads to starvation and disease; disease epidemics serve a purpose by removing the weakest animals. Wolves learned to work together in size-limited groups to maximize their hunting success.

Darwin's famous concept "survival of the fittest" literally means that some of the animals in a population must die before they reach reproductive age in order to maintain a healthy population.

Today, of course, we don't want *our* puppies to be the ones who get culled by Mother Nature. To prevent that, we need to put them on the right path to greater health and fitness. But doing so will challenge many of the most cherished concepts of the medical establishment as well as the pet food industry.

Healthy dogs eating a balanced raw diet are much less susceptible to parasites and infectious diseases. However, raw meat itself can carry parasitic cysts and larvae. Freezing kills most, but not all, of these. In addition, you can assume that all raw meat — even from the grocery store — is contaminated with bacteria: some harmful and some benign. (See Chapter 7 for more about safely preparing a raw diet.) Regular fecal exams will help ensure that your dog's immune system is functioning properly and help prevent internal parasites from gaining a foothold.

FLEAS

Fleas were no doubt a fact of life for Paleo Dogs — they've been around since the first mammals appeared on Earth. However, there were many things that helped protect them from fleas. There were organisms such as beneficial nematodes (worms) that feed on eggs and larvae, and wild-growing medicinal herbs that could be rolled in or nibbled. Our dogs' ancestors were their own herbalists!

But our devotion to the natural dog doesn't have to include putting up with

Saying that parasites are the problem is like saying that "flies cause garbage" just because the two are found together. It is the unhealthy state of the animal that attracts the parasites, just like garbage attracts flies.

In the original Paleo Dogs, health was passed on genetically and epigenetically, so that each generation was at least as healthy as the last. Mankind's interference has undone what Nature did so brilliantly. Now we need to put it back right!

blood-sucking parasites — not to mention the many dangerous diseases they can carry.

First, let's be clear about some of today's flea and tick protection options. For example, flea collars don't work — no matter whether they are herbal or insecticidal. The ones you can get at the store or from your veterinarian contain concentrated toxic chemicals, and the herbal ones are simply annoying to dogs' highly developed sense of smell. Topical (spot-on) flea preventives can also cause serious adverse effects in dogs.

Fighting Fleas

If you're in a flea-endemic area (which is most of the planet), you'll need to take a truly holistic approach; but recognize that this is war! Fleas are tough, dangerous parasites that are not easy to eliminate. Like all parasites, they adapt. All kinds of parasistes can outsmart us genetically by becoming resistant to the products we use to get rid of them, and they can pass these genes along to their progeny (vertical transmission) and in some cases to all of their friends (horizontal transmission) as well.

Fleas are attracted to darkness, warmth, movement, and rhythmic vibrations from feet or paws. In other words, they're attracted to everything about your dog! You not only need to protect your dog but also to root out and kill fleas and larvae hiding in carpets and yards. Even apartment-living dogs can get fleas, which travel in on shoes and clothing. Having everyone remove their shoes at your front door keeps out not only fleas but also other germs, as well as plain old dirt.

Adult fleas spend most of their time on the dog, where they feed on blood several times a day. However, flea eggs are slippery — they quickly fall off the dog and onto the dog's resting areas, floors, rugs, bedding, and furniture. The eggs hatch and go through several intermediate stages before emerging as adults in as little as 2 weeks, but they may remain dormant for months. Reinfestation is a very common and very frustrating phenomenon!

To get rid of fleas, you must take a three-pronged approach and treat the dog, the house, and the yard.

On Your Dog

Use an ultrafine flea comb daily on dogs with amenable coats. The neck, tummy, and base of the tail are favorite flea hangouts. Have a glass full of warm, soapy water at hand to drown any fleas you catch in the comb.

Bathing your dog will drown a lot of fleas, but soap up around the ears and neck first to keep them from rushing up to the dog's head and face. The herb erigeron (fleabane), found in some herbal shampoos, will help kill fleas (see Resources on page 522). Too-frequent bathing or harsh soaps can dry the skin, so use caution.

In Your Home

Floor and carpet treatments such as diatomaceous earth (the fossilized shells of one-celled organisms called diatoms) and boric acid-derived powders will kill flea larvae, primarily through desiccation (drying). You can treat your home with a product containing borates or hire an exterminator like Fleabusters or Flea Stoppers. If you have a serious flea problem, it's worth paying professionals since they guarantee their work.

Vacuuming is very effective against flea eggs and might even catch a few adults. To keep them from hatching or escaping, carefully apply flea spray into the vacuum bag or container and immediately discard the bag or empty the canister when you're done.

Wash bedding (whatever the dog sleeps on) at least weekly. Putting a towel or fleece in favored areas will help confine the pests. Pick it up by the corners to prevent flea eggs from falling out.

In the Yard

Beneficial, predatory nematodes eat flea eggs and will help control flea populations outdoors.

Garden-grade diatomaceous earth will cut and desiccate flea larvae and eggs. Spread the powder liberally on the ground throughout areas under shrubs, decks, and other cool, shady spots where animals (such as raccoons, skunks, and outdoor and feral cats) are most likely to hang out.

TICKS

Ticks are seasonal in most of the United States. The greatest risk is to dogs who get into tall grass, brush, or forested areas, so keep your lawn cut short and your yard neat and well trimmed. You can use a safe herbal repellent spray for walks, hikes, and trips to the park, but still check your dog frequently for ticks, which like to hang out in and around the ears, groin, and armpits, between the toes, and in any skin folds. A tick may attach and feed for several days, but it's important to get rid of them promptly: hopefully before they attach, but at least before they can transmit disease (which may take as little as a few hours).

HEARTWORMS

Heartworms are transmitted by mosquitoes. Tiny heartworm larvae, called microfilaria, circulate in the blood and are sucked up by the bug when it feeds on an infected host animal; for heartworms, their natural host is the dog. Once inside the mosquito, the larvae go through several stages before they can infect another dog. For that to occur, outside temperatures must remain above 57°F, day and night, for a minimum of 8 days. The warmer the temperature, the faster the larvae will mature. If the temperature drops below that critical level, development will stop, but the microfilaria don't die — development will restart at the same point when the weather warms back up. Larvae reach their infective stage in 8 to 30 days (the latter being the entire life span of the average mosquito).

In dogs, the microfilaria migrate to the heart, and over the next 6 to 7 months, they develop into adult worms and reproduce. The next mosquito that bites the dog will suck up the tiny microfilaria and repeat the cycle.

Except for the warmest parts of the United States (like southern Texas and southern Florida), heartworms are a completely seasonal problem. There is no reason to give heartworm medicine to most pets year-round. In many areas of the country, such warm temperatures simply don't exist for most of the year, and sustained warm temperatures don't occur until at least June. Within 150 miles of the Gulf Coast, heartworm risk exists 9 months out of the year. In the rest of the country, heartworm transmission is possible between 3 and 7 months out of the year. Hawaii and Alaska have each had a few cases of canine heartworm, but the incidence in those states is relatively low.

Several drugs on the market kill microfilaria in the blood, so the worms cannot grow and reproduce. While the drugmakers insist that every dog (and cat) needs year-round protection, experts recommend using them *only* during the season when transmission of heartworm is possible.[9] While these drugs are fairly safe and effective, potential side effects include depression and/or lethargy, vomiting, tremors, ataxia (balance problems or unsteady walk), blindness, anorexia, diarrhea, convulsions, weakness and hypersalivation, and contact allergy.

A serious and growing problem is the resistance of heartworms to these drugs.[10] By unnecessarily blasting pets with these chemicals, we are creating super-worms that will be able to survive and grow even in animals on heartworm preventives. As with all cases of resistance, the correct response is to reduce the use of the drug and to reserve it only for when it is absolutely necessary. Unfortunately, the veterinary profession and drug industry continue to call for *all* pets to be on medications *all* year-round. That's bad science, and it's bad policy.

How to Keep Bad Bugs Away

Any dog who goes outside is exposed to pests, but the risk is much higher for dogs who live most of their lives outdoors. Fleas, ticks, and mosquitoes are vectors (carriers) of many diseases, including borreliosis (Lyme disease), ehrlichiosis, heartworms, bubonic plague, and tapeworms. To reduce the risks, be sure to clean out any areas of standing water in your yard (and encourage neighbors to do the same). Mosquitoes can successfully breed in less than a bottle cap's worth of water, so be vigilant. Before your dog heads outside, spritz him with an herbal mosquito repellent. The herbs neem, lemongrass, and catnip, for example, have good insect repellent properties. Keep pets in at dawn and dusk, the mosquitoes' most active time. Always check your dog for ticks after a visit to prime tick habitat, such as long grass, brush, and forested areas.

ELECTROMAGNETIC FIELDS

Electromagnetic fields (EMFs) are invisible lines of force that surround electrical cables as well as electronic devices that we all use daily; they relate to voltage (the amount of power), and their effects also depend on frequency. Magnetic fields result from the flow of current; they stop once the current ceases. Electric fields, on the other hand, are present even when the equipment is switched off, if it is still plugged in. Cordless phones, cellphones, radios, microwave ovens, televisions, hair dryers, lights, refrigerators, and vacuum cleaners all produce EMFs. Research suggests that EMFs — particularly from cellphones (which use microwaves)[11] — may be linked to cancer.[12]

Electric fields are weakened or shielded by trees, buildings, and other objects. Magnetic fields pass through most materials and are more difficult to block.

Both electric and magnetic fields drop off as the distance from the source increases, so it's relatively simple to protect your dog from household EMF sources: Power off electrical devices when not in use, put your cellphone on airplane mode (so it doesn't constantly signal the towers), use battery-powered devices instead of electronics near sleeping areas, and keep the dog out of the kitchen! You may also wish to have your home electrical system checked for problems such as ungrounded outlets. Good old aluminum foil also blocks EMFs, so if you have outlets or appliances that are a particular problem, you've got a handy and cheap solution.

Underground electromagnetic fields, also

called geopathic stress zones, may also affect dogs as well as people. [13]

Blocking EMFs from power lines, cellphone towers, "smart" utility meters, solar flares, airport scanners, and other environmental sources isn't as easy, but it's possible. For a small device, shielding with aluminum foil or some other metal enclosure is one option; check online for various fabrics and other shielding materials and options.

CHAPTER 6
VACCINATION AND THE
IMMUNE SYSTEM

"My veterinarian insisted on vaccinating my dog." "I got a postcard in the mail, so I just did what the vet told me to do." "I didn't know, so I let the tech vaccinate him."

Sound familiar? Vaccinations are still a deeply ingrained part of veterinary medicine. Despite 2 decades of debate and numerous rounds of updated vaccine guidelines from veterinary associations and teaching hospitals, many vets still have not changed their vaccine protocols. This is especially true of large corporate chains of veterinary hospitals.

So what do you do when you get that postcard or email? First, understand that these notices are automatically generated by a computer and do not constitute a mandate. Yes, your dog should have an annual checkup, but vaccines are an entirely separate issue.

Those of us who try to educate people on

the need to make informed decisions about pet vaccination are often vilified as if we were coming out against Mom and her apple pie! Nonetheless, if you are to create a true Paleo Dog Lifestyle for your best friend, caution about vaccines is certainly essential.

If, after carefully considering the risks versus possible benefits, you have had, or plan to have, your dog vaccinated, steps can be taken to minimize the risk of both immediate and long-term adverse health consequences.

SHOULD YOU VACCINATE YOUR DOG?

Newborn puppies are initially protected against disease by maternal immunity that they get from their mother the first few times they suckle. Mom's "first milk," or colostrum, contains antibodies to diseases the mother has been exposed to. For the first 12 to 18 hours of their lives, puppies can absorb these maternal antibodies from their intestines directly into the bloodstream. These antibodies persist for several weeks. This made good evolutionary sense for the original Paleo Puppies, because maternal antibodies were active at the time when the pups emerged from the den and were introduced to the other members of their pack, as well as the local environment.

If a puppy is exposed to a disease for which maternal antibodies are present, those antibodies destroy the organisms and protect the puppy.

Ancient Paleo Dogs were never vaccinated. The environment served to cull the weak from the strong, often through diseases and parasites that occurred early in life. Nature is brutal but efficient. Using our time machine, we can watch the stronger Paleo Puppies nudging out the weaker ones for more than their share of milk, regurgitated food, or fresh kills. These pups grew bigger, developed faster, and played more aggressively — and they survived. And because they did, their species survived, and continues to thrive today.

In Paleo times, puppy mortality may have occasionally been very high. In recent history, researchers have documented the progress of several contagious diseases among the wolves reintroduced to Yellowstone National Park in 1995. While the wolves enjoyed huge population increases during their first few years in the park, later outbreaks of canine distemper killed so many pups that the entire wolf population decreased.[1]

If Paleo Pups survived exposure to infectious diseases during their first, most vulnerable months of life, they gained acquired immunity (antibodies and memory cells) that protected them for life.

Again, we can look to the Yellowstone wolves for clues as to how early Paleo Dogs triumphed over infectious diseases. Canine parvovirus is ubiquitous in the environment, where virus particles can live for many years — even in the wild backcountry of the park. All wolves are likely exposed to it; and indeed, nearly all tested wolves were positive for antibodies to parvovirus by the time they were 6 to 9 months old. The presence of parvo does not appear to affect population numbers. The same is true for canine adenovirus; wolves universally showed evidence of exposure to the disease, but there were no known illnesses.

Vaccination is a highly controversial subject. While certain vaccinations may be justified, overvaccination is extremely harmful. Veterinarians recommend multiple vaccines for puppies, and some or all of these vaccines are typically repeated at intervals throughout the dog's life.

The goal of vaccination is to stimulate the immune system to produce antibodies against a particular disease. It turns out that many viral vaccines are so good at this that they don't need to be boosted every year, or every 3 years, or perhaps at all. Even if circulating antibodies were to decrease, memory cells would most likely provide good protection.

A usually unmentioned purpose of vaccines is not to protect your particular animal against disease (although they are supposed to do that, too) but rather to establish immunity in enough animals so that if a disease does break out, there will not be enough susceptible animals to sustain an epidemic. This is called herd immunity. Broad population immunity through vaccination has prevented the major outbreaks of parvo and distemper that used to be common.

But now, because more and more people are *not* getting their animals vaccinated at all, herd immunity is weakening in many areas. Recent outbreaks of distemper in dogs are causing concern. In some cases, no vaccines may be just as dangerous as too many. Most vets still recommend that puppies get vaccinated for at least parvo and distemper. However, given what we know about the immune system, the idea of booster vaccines needs a deeper examination.

Maternal antibodies are the reason for various puppy vaccination schedules. Vaccinating while maternal antibodies are active is useless: Antibodies destroy the pathogen, and the puppy doesn't produce any antibodies of its own. After maternal antibodies break down, the puppy is completely susceptible. Unfortunately, the strength of immunity and length of time maternal antibodies persist vary greatly, so most veterinarians recommend a vaccine *series* to bridge possible gaps and to make sure the puppy's own immune response is adequate.

The truth is that there was never any science showing the need for annual vaccines. Dr. Ron Schultz and Dr. Tom R. Phillips, of the department of pathobiological sciences at the University of Wisconsin School of Veterinary Medicine, said:

A practice that was started many years ago and that lacks scientific validity or verification is annual revaccinations. Almost without exception there is no immunologic requirement for annual revaccination. Immunity to viruses persists for years or for the life of the animal. . . . Furthermore, revaccination with most viral vaccines fails to stimulate an anamnestic (secondary) response as a result of interference by existing antibody (similar to maternal antibody interference).[2]

In plain English, this means that there is no valid scientific reason to vaccinate pets every year; the basic principles of immunology actually argue against it. Booster vaccines do not improve immunity, but they do increase the risk of adverse effects.

There is just as much science underlying the current recommendation of boostering core vaccines every 3 years — by which we mean *none.* In fact, recent guidelines from the American Animal Hospital Association (AAHA) acknowledge that the distemper and parvo vaccines provide *at least* 5 years of protection, and probably protection for life in most dogs.[3]

Today, we know that vaccines are not harmless; they should be considered a medical procedure like any other, with both risks and benefits. The potential risks and benefits of each and every vaccine your vet recommends should be considered for your dog individually, based on age, breed, health, lifestyle, and history.

Vaccine Safety

Millions of dogs are vaccinated every year. Most of them appear to come through it just fine. Unless symptoms occur within 72 hours after vaccination, allopathic veterinarians and vaccine makers are quite comfortable denying any and all connection between diseases (especially chronic diseases) and vaccines. But the science is not on their side. Holistic veterinarians understand that vaccine-related diseases can occur at any time during the life of our dogs, whether or not symptoms are seen close to the time of vaccination.

The goal of vaccination is to produce antibodies, the blood proteins that attack and destroy invading organisms. We want the body to produce antibodies against the disease being vaccinated against. However, the vaccine manufacturing process results in the body making antibodies not just to the pathogen but also to a wide variety of components in the vaccine.

Most vaccines are produced using a culture medium such as eggs, blood serum, or certain types of cells. The organisms are

163

grown in these nutritious cultures, and then filtered and manufactured into vaccines. Here's the problem: While the filters are small enough to keep out whole cells, both the intended virus particles and a variety of *unintended* proteins from the culture medium will end up in the final product. When that product is injected, the body doesn't distinguish among these many ingredients; it makes antibodies to the stray proteins as well as to the pathogenic organism.

Studies at Purdue University showed that canine vaccines grown in calf serum caused antibodies to be made to many things, including red blood cells, thyroid tissue, DNA, and connective tissue proteins, among many others. Unfortunately, bovine proteins are so similar to dog proteins that the antibodies react to the puppies' own tissue as well — this is an autoimmune reaction ("auto" means "self"). Every vaccinated puppy developed multiple autoantibodies, and every additional booster produced even more. Autoantibodies made by the puppies' immune systems included the thyroid gland, red blood cells, collagen (the major structural protein in the body), cardiolipin (found in heart valves), and even their own DNA.[4] So far, there is a strong indication that vaccines are linked to canine hypothyroidism[5] and canine diabetes.[6] Researchers have stated point-blank that autoimmune disease is an *inevitable consequence* of repeated vaccination.[7]

One reason why vaccines can have such deleterious effects is the fact that they are injected. Most of the diseases we vaccinate against are acquired in nature through direct contact between the dog's respiratory, gastrointestinal, or urogenital system and the disease organism. These systems have their own defenses; and in particular, they produce a type of antibody called immunoglobulin A (IgA). This anti-body is secreted by immune cells living in the mucous membranes that have direct contact with the outside world (e.g., eyes, nose, mouth, lungs, intestines, and urethra), providing a rapid, local response that kills most invading organisms. Injecting the vaccine puts those organisms (whether modified or killed) into direct contact with the bloodstream, bypassing IgA and creating a type of invasion that is never encountered in nature. The immune system will still make the other antibodies it would normally make, and which generate vaccine-induced immunity.

Intranasal vaccines are becoming more popular, although at this time they are only available against a few pathogens, such as those that cause kennel cough. Because they are entering the body through the natural route, intranasal vaccines are much safer and do not appear to create the kind of long-term damage we see with injectable vaccines. We look forward to the time when they will be available for more dangerous viruses, such as parvo and distemper.

Vaccine Efficacy

Vaccine advocates (aka pharmaceutical companies and people who get paid by pharmaceutical companies) claim that vaccines have reduced or eliminated a wide variety of diseases in both humans and animals, in countries or continents or the whole world. Smallpox is a favorite example. However, the incidence of smallpox was already on the wane when the vaccine was introduced, mainly because of broad social improvements, particularly in sanitation and nutrition education. The same holds true for many other communicable diseases: They were naturally declining before vaccines came along.[8]

The reality is that the incidence of smallpox, polio, and other diseases *increased* after the introduction of vaccines. In countries that did not adopt the polio vaccine, for example, the polio "epidemic" didn't keep going; it died on its own. Today, most cases of polio are *caused by the polio vaccine.*[9] For diseases like measles and whooping cough, between 50 and 90 percent of the people who contract these diseases today *are fully vaccinated,* which certainly casts doubt on vaccines' effectiveness.

Humans are heavily vaccinated in infancy and childhood, and boosters are not repeated more than a few times in our much longer lives (if at all). In contrast, dogs are vaccinated several times as puppies and then annually or even more often; kennel cough (*Bordetella*) and leptospirosis vaccines are often recommended every 6 months.

Unfortunately for us and our dogs, vaccines are the fastest-growing segment of the pharmaceutical industry. Currently, there are more than 300 vaccines in development for humans, including those against cancer, meningitis, antibiotic-resistant "superbugs," malaria, nicotine, methamphetamines, and of course, AIDS.[10]

The USDA, not the FDA, regulates animal vaccines. According to evidence-based medicine advocate David Ramey, DVM, the USDA "merely requires that vaccines be shown to be safe and pure, with a 'reasonable expectation' of efficacy prior to their release; however, the clinical need (relevancy) or usefulness (applicability) of a particular vaccine may not necessarily be assured by the licensing process."[11]

The worst risks associated with vaccination are due to *over*vaccination. Some vaccines offer protection to young puppies from devastating, potentially fatal diseases like parvo and distemper, as well as rabies (rabies vaccination is required by law in most places). These are called "core" vaccines, and they are universally recommended by veterinarians. However, adult dogs do not need annual, biannual, or even triennial boosters for puppy diseases, and with rare exception, they don't need most other vaccines, such as rattlesnake venom, melanoma, Giardia, leptospirosis, Lyme disease, periodontal (gum) disease, coronavirus, and canine influenza.

Rabies Vaccines

Even though the rabies vaccine is legally required every 3 years by all 50 states (or even more often by some cities and counties), it probably protects against this serious public health threat for a much longer period.[12] Until now, nobody has challenged animals with the rabies virus over a longer period of time; however, the Rabies Challenge Fund is currently performing this much-needed research. (Please support the group's efforts at www.rabieschallengefund.org.)

If your dog has had a bad reaction to a previous rabies vaccine or if your dog is not completely healthy, you may be able to get an exemption letter from your veterinarian. In most jurisdictions, this will allow you to keep your dog's license current without the vaccine.

Most places legally require one puppy vaccine, a booster 1 year later, and a revaccination every 1 to 3 years thereafter. If possible, wait until your puppy is 6 months old for the first vaccine to allow the immune system to mature. Unfortunately, many states require the first rabies vaccine at 12 weeks of age, and there could be legal consequences if your unvaccinated puppy bites someone. Laws may require (and public health officials recommend) that adult dogs with an unknown vaccine history should receive one rabies vaccine and a booster 1 year later, and thereafter get revaccinated as required by law.

IF YOU DECIDE TO VACCINATE
Make sure your dog is as healthy as possible at the time of vaccination. Do not al-

low any other treatment to take place at the same time, including any medication (a dog needing medication is not healthy and therefore not eligible for vaccination), surgery, teeth cleaning, or even bathing.

All canine vaccines explicitly state on the label "For Use in Healthy Dogs Only." Do not vaccinate geriatric, sick, debilitated, medicated, or immune-compromised dogs.

Always use vaccines with the fewest antigens. Avoid products like "5-way" or "7-way" vaccines that include coronavirus, *Leptospira* and Lyme bacteria, parainfluenza, or other unnecessary additions.

Whatever vaccines you and your veterinarian agree on, avoid the common practice of giving multiple, simultaneous vaccines. Research indicates that this is not only less efficacious but is also far more likely to produce unacceptable side effects, especially in small dogs.[13] Vaccines should be spaced. Also avoid vaccinating for 30 days prior to and during estrus, pregnancy, or lactation.

We believe that the best defense against any disease is a healthy immune system, but how many dogs today are truly healthy? Research in the new field of epigenetics shows that many factors experienced by your dog's ancestors — even stress — can have a negative effect for generations.

Nevertheless, if you forgo some or all vaccines, you may face some tough questions: Will my veterinarian continue to examine and treat my dog? (A few won't.) Will boarding kennels or groomers allow my dog in their facilities? (Many won't.)

Be cautious when going to a new veterinarian (especially for an emergency) whose vaccine policy you may not know. A vet's belief system — and therefore clinic policy — can be so ingrained that if your pet is taken from your control (e.g., for a nail trim, a blood draw, or another procedure), one or more vaccines might automatically be given. We know cases where a vet or a technician vaccinated a pet without permission — and it only came to light because a charge for vaccination was added to the bill! Make sure it is written in your chart that your dog cannot be vaccinated without your written consent. Also, make it clear that you do not want topical flea products or any other medications administered without your explicit permission.

It is important to understand that no vaccine is 100 percent effective, and that vaccine "breaks" (failure to induce immunity) do occur. There may be a genetic component as to whether a puppy or adult dog will respond to vaccination at all.

If you choose to vaccinate a young puppy, be aware that vaccine immunity takes at least 10 to 14 days to reach its full effect. Parvovirus is persistent everywhere in the environment, so it's essential to avoid dog parks, puppy classes, and socializing with unknown dogs until your puppy is protected. For unvaccinated puppies, similar care is advised. Seek supportive veterinary care at the first sign of illness in a puppy.

If you want to protect an adult dog with an unknown vaccination history, one distemper-parvo vaccine after 16 weeks of age provides immunity for many years, and probably for life in most dogs.[14]

Some breeders will start vaccinating puppies at 2 weeks of age and revaccinate every 2 weeks until the puppies go to their new homes, even when the parents are themselves fully vaccinated. There is no justification for this practice, because the mother's maternal antibodies prevent the puppies from developing their own immunity. There's plenty that can go wrong with repeatedly overwhelming an infant's vulnerable immune system with multiple vaccines.

Here are some suggestions on how to prevent adverse effects from injectable vaccines, as well as intranasal ones.[15] Please be aware that vaccine reactions often do not happen immediately. Plan ahead if you can, and be prepared! Do clear the use of these precautionary measures with your veterinarian, who will hopefully be open to alternative treatments. If not, consider finding a new veterinarian who is willing to work with you. Remember, your veterinarian *works for you,* and the relationship created between you is deemed a personal service contract. You have every right to go elsewhere until you find someone whose knowledge and experience is a good fit with your own.

The following are suggestions to help reduce side effects that can arise from vaccination. (See Resources on page 511 for specific product recommendations.)

One hour before vaccination: Give by mouth (1) a dose of marine-source omega-3 fatty acids (see Appendix A on page 419 and Resources on page 529) and (2) a dose of antioxidants, such as curcumin, quercetin, astaxanthin, vitamin C, and vitamin E. Antioxidants have anti-inflammatory properties that may help prevent vaccine reactions. Curcumin (the active compound in turmeric) and quercetin in particular have been found to block the ability of the adjuvants in killed vaccines to trigger a chronic immune reaction. Vitamin E (in a natural form that is high in gamma-E) may help dampen the immune reactions and may also reduce several of the inflammatory cytokines (messenger proteins). Vitamin C is also a very potent anti-inflammatory; be sure to use a non-GMO, buffered form (such as sodium or calcium ascorbate), not ascorbic acid (which is usually synthetic; see Resources). Antioxidants work better in combination than singly.

Immediately before vaccination (or as close as possible): Give a calcium supplement. It needs to contact the mucous membranes of the mouth, so place it in your dog's mouth; even a tiny bit of a calcium tablet will work.

After the vaccine is injected: Immediately apply a cold pack or ice pack to the injection site. This will inhibit bloodflow to the area and keep the vaccine ingredients from spreading into the blood and surrounding tissues. This is especially important for vaccines that contain adjuvants. Take your own ice pack with you if possible, or request one before the vaccination is given (most vets have lots of these little packs laying around).

174

Give a dose of the homeopathic *Thuja occidentalis* 30C immediately after vaccination (within 2 hours), and give another dose every 12 hours for a total of three doses (more is not necessary and may negate the benefits). Homeopathy is able to head off many adverse vaccine effects, including those that may appear months or even years later. If you are working with a veterinary homeopath, check to make sure this is the appropriate remedy (there are others that may be better for your particular dog). In the absence of specific instructions from a homeopathic veterinarian, *Thuja* is the most broadly applicable remedy.

Topical magnesium chloride can be beneficial for cellular stress from chemical insults. Magnesium chloride bath flakes, gels, lotions, and oils are excellent topical choices. If administering oral magnesium, check the dose with your veterinarian.

Green supplement: Mix a little organic parsley and organic celery, which can be pureed in a blender with a little water, and add it to your dog food for a week or two after vaccination. Parsley is very high in a flavonoid called apigenin, and celery is high in luteolin. Both are very potent in inhibiting autoimmune diseases.

NOTE: Do *not* give your dog immune-stimulating supplements, such as mushroom extracts, whey protein powders, echinacea, or beta-glucans right after vaccinating.

Avoid all mercury-containing seafood and other sources of mercury, such as inexpensive, unpurified fish oil, as this heavy metal is a very powerful inducer of autoimmunity and is known to make people and pets more susceptible to viral infections. Mercury is still found in many vaccines. Do not feed your dog tuna, salmon, or other predatory or carnivorous fish, or fish oils from these sources. The older and larger the fish, the more toxins will have accumulated in its body; and those toxins are delivered unchanged, via pet food, to your dog.

After consulting with your team of experts, keep a positive mindset about the informed choices you make for yourself, your children, and your pets. Intention and expectation do play a role in creating a healthy future for you and your family.

Helping Previously Vaccinated Dogs
Some dogs may not appear to be negatively affected by vaccination. Those who are affected typically show subtle signs of energy imbalance such as those mentioned in Chapter 1 or they may become obviously ill with any of several ailments. It's best to

contact a holistic practitioner as soon as you see a problem.

Even if you become certain that vaccination made your animal ill, please don't feel guilty. Remember that you did your best, based on the advice of experts — the veterinarians to whom you entrusted the care of your animal; and they, too, were doing what they were taught was appropriate, or what their clinic required. Many veterinarians are still in denial about the potential harm vaccines can cause. The evidence of their own eyes supports them — in most cases, there is no quick or obvious cause-and-effect relationship of vaccines to chronic disease.

Homeopathy and flower essences are especially good therapies for vaccinosis (see Resources on page 514). While they're not strictly Paleo therapies, they may be needed to treat this very non-Paleo disease.

Nosodes

You may have heard of "homeopathic vaccines" or "vaccine alternatives." These terms refer to a type of remedy called a nosode: a homeopathically prepared remedy made from diseased tissues or discharges from an infected but unvaccinated and untreated animal.

Nosodes are given to unvaccinated animals to prevent a disease or to treat a set of symptoms resembling that disease. They have been particularly useful in cases of rapidly spreading infectious diseases like kennel cough. Unlike vaccines, nosodes are said to be safe; there is evidence for their efficacy when used properly. Many homeopathically trained veterinarians feel that they are highly effective and valuable tools in the prevention of various infectious diseases. If you want to explore the possibility of using nosodes for your dog, please consult with a homeopathic veterinarian (see Resources on page 511).

Titer Testing

To determine whether your dog needs a booster vaccine, you can have an antibody titer (a measurement of how many active antibodies a dog has against any particular disease) done using a blood sample. Antibodies to many diseases may have formed as a result of either vaccination or natural exposure. There are titers for many diseases, but not all, and the titer for each disease must be performed individually. Unfortunately, there is no consensus on what level of antibodies (what titer) is needed for an individual's protection — although a very high titer most likely indicates adequate immunity. If you choose to have titers run on your dog, it is very important to ask for *vaccine-related immunity* and to start at low dilutions when ordering the tests; otherwise, the lab will test for the active virus, and the results will be distorted. Keep in mind that a titer is only a snapshot of one part of the immune system and may not give an accurate picture of the dog's actual risk of disease.

THE PARADIGM OF FEAR

Our present medical and veterinary systems are built entirely on fear: fear of disease, fear of injury, fear of cancer, fear of death. It turns out that fear is a very handy tool for getting people to do what you want.

In veterinary school, we were actually taught to always give clients the worst-case scenario, because if you were right and the animal got sicker, the family was prepared; and if you were wrong and the animal got better (often despite your treatment), you would look like a genius! Unfortunately, fear can also be used to manipulate people into getting vaccinations and preventive medicines that their dog doesn't need, or expensive surgeries or other treatments that may not be effective.

Fear is a stressful and unhealthy state.

When an animal is frightened, its sympathetic nervous system is activated, producing a cascade of chemical messengers and hormones like adrenaline that prepare the body for "fight or flight." If the stress is not relieved, the body will shift from the adrenaline-fueled "I'm about to die" response to a more chronic one in which it produces constantly elevated levels of cortisol.

Cortisol is part of a regulatory system that affects the circulatory system, the nervous system, and the immune system. In particular, it suppresses the immune response, which makes the body more susceptible to infection. It also increases appetite and thirst; weight gain is a common side effect.

Our dogs' Paleo ancestors knew what responding to life-and-death events meant. They had a real need for an instantaneous fight-or-flight reflex. Today, just the fact of modern living — with its constant light, noise, and stimulation — keeps us and our dogs in a chronic state of stress that ultimately takes a terrible toll on our bodies.

At any given moment, billions of bacteria are living on a dog's skin and coat, in its mouth, and in its digestive tract. Microbes that coexist with the dog in a mutually beneficial (symbiotic) relationship are known as symbionts. The immune system's job is to recognize nonsymbionts and to kill or otherwise effectively eliminate them. This process occurs thousands of times per day.

Today, as a result of our overuse of antibiotics, particularly in livestock, bacteria have developed multiple-drug resistance, resulting in superbugs like the "flesh-eating" bacteria (methicillin-resistant *Staphylococcus aureus,* or MRSA). And once one bacterium figures it out, it can transfer that resistance to not only all of its relatives but also to completely different species of bacteria. And it doesn't stop with bacteria; as we discussed in Chapter 5, there's evidence that heartworms are developing resistance to the drugs we use to prevent them.

You can clearly see that we haven't achieved much by declaring war on germs.

MAINTAINING OPTIMAL HEALTH

Acute diseases, such as distemper, are often accompanied by a high fever, which is a primary defense mechanism: Many viruses cannot survive at even slightly higher temperatures. If all goes well, the fever breaks and recovery can proceed. The immune system has also identified the organism involved and is prepared to fight it more effectively in the future.

Both humans and dogs may develop the same symptoms, such as a cough and mucus. However, these are usually secondary to the first problem: an unhealthy terrain. This simply means that the body is moved out of balance (homeostasis) by factors such as an unhealthy lifestyle, stress, drugs, chemicals, and vaccination. These stressors overload our immune systems, thereby making us vulnerable to opportunistic germs, such as viruses, fungi, and bacteria.

To become Paleo Dogs, our dogs need to have their internal and external terrain detoxified, nourished, nurtured, and loved to regain and maintain health.

When we are in optimum health, our friendly and so-called unfriendly bacteria coexist with us, and function within their own system of checks and balances. The immune system monitors normal bacterial populations, as well as invading organisms, and eliminates threats. This process occurs thousands of times per day. But it is not the "invasion" of microbes that leads to infection; it is the compromise of the body — the terrain — that allows this to occur.

A big problem in veterinary medicine today is the fear of pathogens. Vaccinations and antibiotics and all kinds of toxic treatments are used to combat germs. But animals evolved with microbes, and Mother Nature created the immune system for the purpose of dealing with them. Persistently seeking a vaccine for every new germ and a drug for each symptom keeps us chained to an endless cycle of dysfunctional medical care.

We think it's time we give our Paleo Dogs' immune systems more credit and dispel their frailty as a medical myth. We can simply expand our belief systems to allow for a better understanding of the relationship between all living things and microbes. After all, they are here to stay.

PART III
GOING PALEO

CHAPTER 7
FEEDING THE PALEO DOG

Eating right is the key to good health and longevity for people, and it's the same for our dogs. Vitality, contentment, and zest for life come from within. They spring from a body and brain that are fully supplied with essential nutrients in the right form. The best nutrition provides the dog's body what it needs without burdening the body with indigestible waste, chemical additives, or other harmful substances. To live out the longest life possible in optimum health, your dog needs to eat well. In this chapter, we'll show you exactly how to accomplish that.

Many people become squeamish when they first hear about feeding their dogs raw meat, but this would be your dog's choice in the wild. Now that dogs live with us in our homes, we have removed that choice and forced them to eat things they would never eat in the natural world.

The presence of pathogens associated with

raw meat demands respect as well as safe meat handling procedures (by humans, that is). The dog itself has many natural defenses, including the following:

- The mucous membranes and the mouth's resident bacteria provide a physical barrier.
- Saliva contains lysozymes that can break down the cell walls of invading organisms.
- Many pathogens are destroyed by the dog's very acidic stomach juices. Food in the stomach is churned around by the powerful stomach muscles, which help to expose every surface of the food to hydrochloric acid.
- The dog's short small intestine pushes food through relatively quickly, so invaders cannot get a foothold.[1] (The dog's body length–to–digestive tract ratio is only 1:6, compared with 1:12 for the horse and 1:20 for the cow.)[2]
- The small intestine is where most digestion takes place, and it is bristling with defenses. As with the rest of the digestive system, a mucous membrane is the first physical barrier, in which resident probiotic bacteria stand ready to defend their home. You may have

heard that 70 to 80 percent of the immune system is in the digestive tract, and it's found in the top layer of tissue, where a hefty population of white blood cells lives, many of them concentrated into strongholds called Peyer's patches.

- If pathogens do make it into the bloodstream, they're immediately taken to the liver — the body's main detoxifying organ — which is itself abundantly supplied with immune cells. In fact, all blood leaving the digestive organs is routed through the liver, so that invaders and all kinds of toxins can be dealt with.
- Finally, the undigested portion of the food passes through the large intestine, where competition from normal resident bacteria protects against the invaders that get there alive.

Freezing raw meat for 72 hours at 0°F (-18°C) kills *Toxoplasma gondii* and *Neospora caninum* cysts.[3] While bacteria aren't affected by freezing, consider this: A mother dog licks the backsides of her puppies, and she ingests what comes out of them for several weeks following their birth! A newborn puppy's gastrointestinal tract is fully loaded with bacteria within 24 hours of birth.[4] Dogs also clean their own bacteria-laden backsides, paws, and bodies for the rest of their lives, so you can appreciate the natural cleansing ability of the dog.

However, depending on the health of your dog, you should proceed cautiously when introducing the homemade Paleo Dog Diet. In the beginning, you may need to cook the meat. Over time, you can cook the meat less and less until you're serving it completely raw. The road to wellness and recovery will depend on shifting the dog's diet as close to nature as possible.

A few dogs may never do well on a strictly Paleo Dog Diet; they seem to need some of the carbohydrates and fiber that their systems have become accustomed to. We recommend taking it one tiny step at a time; if you have any doubts, go back a step or consult your holistic vet. See Chapter 9 for information on potential problems and how to solve them.

THE PAWS SYSTEM: ASSESSING THE QUALITY OF YOUR DOG'S DIET

People feed their dogs in many different ways — some better, others not so good. To help you understand how your current feeding practices affect your dog's health, we'll rank each regime by the Paws System. The best, healthiest food gets a rating of 5 paws, while the least healthful and nutritious gets only 1 paw — or none. Any of these methods will fall somewhat short of the diet that a wild dog chooses for himself, but obviously it's not practical — or safe — for your pet to go hunting!

We understand that, for multiple and/or large dogs, the cost of the food may be a significant issue. If you can only add a little meatball of raw meat a couple of times a week, or feed your dog a home-made dinner just on Sundays, please do it! The benefits of fresh food are impossible to overstate. After all, don't our human physicians advise us to eat more fresh foods? It's not for nothing — fresh foods are loaded with enzymes, antioxidants, and a sort of life force that processed foods completely lack. As they say in politics, "Don't let the perfect be the enemy of the good." A little bit is definitely much better than none!

Wherever you currently fall in the Paws System, do your best to achieve 5 paws, or at least get as far down that road as you can go. Your dog is completely dependent on you to provide a healthy diet. It will be worth every bit of effort to avoid the many health problems associated with the wrong diet, and it will help your dog heal from any problems he has — as well as thwart those that may be brewing deep inside.

5 Paws: The Paleo Dog homemade raw-meat diet. This diet is ideal because you can personally control the quality and amount of every ingredient. Alternatively, you can buy similar commercial low-carb, raw-meat diets in frozen, freeze-dried, and dehydrated varieties, either online or in many specialty pet stores. Raw meat can be lightly sautéed or cooked as an intermediate stage for dogs transitioning to a raw diet, or even as the final stage for dogs who can't have or don't do well on raw meat. Make sure the food is at a safe temperature before feeding, and add digestive enzymes and probiotics just before serving.

4 Paws: Organic or natural canned dog food. A sprinkle of digestive enzymes is a must. To take this diet up a notch, add a little fresh raw or lightly cooked meat to each meal — or whenever you can.

Even a weekly treat of raw meat is far better than none.

3 Paws: Other canned dog food, whether a major brand that is sold by pet food retailers or recommended by veterinarians, or a grocery or discount-store brand. Supplement the food with digestive enzymes, probiotics, and omega-3 fatty acids.

2 Paws: Organic and natural dry dog food. The definition of *natural* is very broad and allows for genetically modified and artificially processed ingredients that most of us would consider completely *un*natural. The term *organic* does have a very strict legal definition. If you are looking for an organic dog food, be sure to read the ingredient list carefully. You might find that every ingredient has the term *organic* in front of it *except* the primary protein. For example, you might see something like: "Organic chicken, organic brown rice, *chicken meal,* organic carrots . . ." Because the "organic chicken" is mostly water, the chicken meal — which is not organic — is the primary protein. If an ingredient doesn't specifically say organic, it isn't.

1 Paw: Other dry dog food, including premium and "veterinary" brands, as well as grocery, discount, and private label brands that are found only within specific store chains.

No Paws: An all-meat or raw-meaty-bones-only diet with no added supplements. This is extremely unbalanced and will cause serious nutritional deficiencies over time.

If you do feed your dog commercial pet food, there are ways to make sure it's as good as it can be. First, realize that there is a great divide between various dry foods. Because of the way they are processed, dry foods must use rendered meals as their major animal-source ingredients. Meat meals do contain higher proportions of protein than meat, since the fat and water have been removed. Because of the processing, no dry food will ever be great, but some are definitely better than others.

Avoid foods containing by-product meal, meat and bone meal, beef and bone meal, and similar ingredients, as well as animal fat (if the ingredient list specifies a fat by name, such as chicken fat, that's okay). These tend to be the least expensive (and thus poorest quality) animal-source ingredients. Meat and bone meal (MBM) is the mammal equivalent to by-product meal (which technically applies only to poultry). Animal fat and meat and bone meal were reported as the ingredients most likely to contain the drug used for euthanasia (sodium pentobarbital) in a study conducted by the FDA.[5]

A named meat or meat meal should be the primary protein source, rather than a cereal like corn gluten meal. Corn and soy, in all forms, must be avoided. Corn has the same glycemic index as a chocolate bar. Corn gluten meal, a high-protein corn extract, is often substituted for more expensive meat ingredients. Its presence in a food clearly indicates a company's preference for economy over nutritional value. Because soybeans are relatively high in protein, they are commonly substituted for animal proteins. Soy and corn are the ingredients most likely to be genetically modified; and in fact, unless the dog food and all of its ingredients are organic, we guarantee that all corn and soy are genetically modified.

Then there are the grain-free diets, which may not be all that much better as an alternative. In most cases, the manufacturer simply substitutes starchy vegetables, like potatoes, sweet potatoes, or green peas, for grains; the carbohydrate content remains too high. And, of course, it's all still processed.

INTRODUCING THE PALEO DOG DIET

You may have decided to make your own dog food for all the reasons we have presented. And you may have performed independent research or perused other books before reading this one. However, most diets and recipes found in pet cookbooks or online are not complete or balanced. Many veterinarians are absolutely against raw and homemade diets of any kind, exactly because they have seen animals that have become very sick from improperly made homemade diets; those are the cases that tend to get published, so veterinarians hear about them and pass their thoughts on to you.

The most serious problems arise from feeding only raw meat or meaty bones as a substitute for commercial dog food. The dog does need a diet based on raw meat, but must also receive supplements that provide all necessary nutrients, including calcium and other minerals, vitamins, healthy fats, enzymes, amino acids, and other trace nutrients.

When wolves make a kill, they consume the meat, of course, but also the organs and

196

glands (which contain different mixes of nutrients), and most important, the blood, which contains a vast array of nutrients and compounds. When livestock and poultry are slaughtered, the first thing removed is the blood, so our dogs cannot get the same nutrition from store-bought meat as they would from meat caught in the wild. Even if you are getting whole rabbits or whole quail directly from the farm, they will not contain that all-important blood.

Feeding only raw chicken necks, backs, wings, or even whole chickens does not constitute a properly prepared raw-meat diet, either, especially because modern livestock and poultry contain a very un-natural meat-to-bone ratio. Meat animals have been bred to produce much more muscle and fat than a rabbit, deer, or other natural canine prey would have. This must be taken into account in balancing your dog's diet, especially if you are using bone-in ground meat or poultry. We have calculated this for you in our recipes.

Many people start out with a decent recipe and the best intentions, but over time, they run out of a supplement and forget to replace it, or they get in the habit of feeding just one kind of meat, or they get off track in some way or another. This is called diet drift, and it is a good way to create nutritional deficiencies or excesses — and consequently serious health problems — for your dog. There is a reason for every ingredient, and deficiencies may not be obvious until it's too late.

We'll be providing the recipes themselves in Chapter 8, but first we want to help you understand some basic concepts.

SWITCHING FOODS

We hope we have convinced you to at least upgrade your dog's diet, even if you're not ready to go all the way to Paleo!

Many dogs are quite amenable to new and different foods. But for others, it takes a bit of strategy to accomplish this goal. And even if they are willing to switch, doing so suddenly isn't always the best idea, as it risks unpleasant tummy upsets. Here are some tips for making this transition.

For dogs who have had food available day and night (free choice), the first step is to go to a timed meal schedule, where you leave the food out for 1 hour in the morning and again for 1 hour in the evening, but put it away the rest of the time. Your dog will not starve to death in 12 hours, or even 14 or 18 hours. The eat-fast-eat schedule is more natural to carnivores; it gives them time to digest between meals, and allows the system to rest. The other big advantage of timed meals is that your dog will be hungry at mealtime, and thus be more willing to try new things. This is particularly helpful when moving away from dry food. Do this for at least a week.

If you are just starting your dog on raw food, it's best to make a gradual switch, even if your dog loves the new food (and especially if he doesn't!). An abrupt change in diet can cause diarrhea, vomiting, and general unwellness. These foods are so different that it will take your dog's system some time to acclimate. Start with no more than 25 percent new food, then 50 percent new and 50 percent old, then 75 percent new and 25 percent old.

Increase portions only slightly or feed another small meal if your dog still acts hungry and wants more. Let him digest what you have fed him. You don't want to overfill the stomach, which may cause vomiting.

The amount of food your dog wants or is willing to eat may vary. We don't always want the same amount of food at the same time every day; and though having a routine is preferable, be aware of factors that may alter your dog's needs and appetite. Feed a bit less than the dry or canned food you are currently feeding, as raw meat and raw bones are much more nutrient dense. Do keep in mind that dogs and puppies — just like us humans — don't always want to eat every meal you serve them and at times are not as hungry. Give them a little flexibility to make their own decisions. But do keep an eye on what goes into their tummies and what comes out the other end! Digestion of raw meat usually takes no more than 4 hours and makes its first appearance in the small intestine in about 20 minutes. Dry food takes between 12 and as long as 24 hours to be processed through the dog's gut. This is more like putrefaction than actual healthy digestion and creates an ideal breeding ground for parasites and bacteria.

OVERCOMING OBSTACLES

Preparing your dog's food at home may seem too daunting for many reasons, but the two most common objections are time and money. We're here to bust these myths and set the record straight!

Obstacle 1: It takes too much time. Many people who are new to this method of feeding worry about how time-consuming the preparation of homemade meals may be. But all you need is a good system, like making large batches and freezing meal-size portions. On average, people who feed their dog a homemade raw diet say it takes about 10 minutes per day. Isn't your dog worth that?

Obstacle 2: It costs too much money. It's true that there are some "start-up costs" for the Paleo Diet, especially for those who switch from buying a giant bag of store-brand kibble to lots of high-quality meats. You need to purchase supplements, and you may want to invest in tools, such as a meat grinder or food processor, to make the job easier (which will, of course, save big over time). But remember that the Paleo Dog Diet is the ultimate preventive health measure. A lifetime of commercial pet food is a virtual guarantee that your dog will develop one or more chronic diseases. The Paleo Dog Diet will save you money on veterinary bills in the long run — as well as give your dog a longer, healthier life.

CALCIUM AND RAW BONES

Bones are quite naturally a part of the Paleo Dog Diet. But before you run off to the butcher, we need to discuss how to add bones to your dog's diet in a safe, reasonable way. While it is true that carnivores have been eating raw prey, bones and all, for more than 40 million years, today's domesticated dogs come in all shapes, sizes, and health conditions. They need to ease into their new role as Paleo Dogs.

Calcium is essential in the dog's diet; it's the most common mineral in the body. It's found not only in bones (although 99 percent of it resides there) but also in the blood and throughout all tissues. Calcium is what enables muscles to contract, the heart to beat, and nerve impulses to travel. If a dog doesn't get enough calcium in his food, his body will leach it from the bones, leading to weakness and brittleness of the skeleton. All-meat diets are notorious for causing severe calcium deficiencies; animals seem fine, right up until the day they break a leg just walking across the living room because their bones have become so depleted.

Conversely, too much calcium, especially in puppies, can cause serious orthopedic abnormalities. Puppies, of course, would get their calcium from their mother's milk — a relatively rich source. Canine milk is higher in fat and protein than cow's milk.

For the modern Paleo Dog, the form that makes the most sense is bone meal, and the safest source is New Zealand, one of very few countries free of mad cow disease and its predecessor, sheep scrapie. Bone meal, as well as calcium supplements containing dolomite or calcium carbonate, are concerning because of their potential contamination with lead. Since the introduction of unleaded gasoline in the 1970s, environmental sources of lead have greatly diminished, but low levels may still be present.[6] Lead toxicity is cumulative and permanent.

Care must be taken to include the right amount of bone meal to achieve the correct ratio of calcium, magnesium, and other minerals to muscle meat, which is high in phosphorus. Too much calcium, especially in puppies, is nearly as bad as not enough.

We also need to acknowledge that many dogs today are starting out already debilitated by generations of kibble, overvaccination, and other aspects of their near ancestors' not-so-Paleo lifestyles. It's best to start out very gently when it comes to bones.

Therefore, a supplement containing bone meal (along with other vitamins and minerals) or plain bone meal from an edible source (not bone meal for the garden) is the safest place to start (see Resources on page 529). Paleo Dogs obtained most of their calcium from their prey's bones, so bone meal is an easy way to accomplish this balance when starting our homemade Paleo

Dog Diet.

After your dog has fully transitioned to the basic recipe, the next step is to add ground raw bones into the food. You can have your butcher grind chicken backs and necks — or even a whole chicken if you wish. Be sure the butcher runs them through the grinder at least three times. You can also purchase your own meat grinder to grind meats and poultry. Be certain that bone chunks are small enough that your dog can handle them easily.

Feeding whole bones may never work for some individual dogs and dog breeds. You need to be the judge of this by looking at the shape of your dog's face and jaw and examining the dentition. The first Paleo Dogs were wolves, which, as adults, had long, powerful jaws with 42 properly spaced, large, healthy teeth. They began to chew on bones as tiny puppies, slowly building up their jaw strength. They grew up burying uneaten parts of their kill and then digging these parts up again for a luscious smelly meal days or even weeks later.

What wolves did *not* have were short noses with 42 small teeth crowded into an even smaller mouth. Many toy breed and brachycephalic (short-nosed) dogs suffer from abnormal dentition that may not be suitable for crunching on bones; and if they have missing or decaying teeth, gnawing bones may be painful. However, even for these dogs, you may eventually be able to cut off one vertebrae from a chicken neck and then pound it with a mallet so the bones inside the muscle tissues break up — all the better for your little dog to handle them.

If your bigger dog has been eating like a Paleo Dog for some time, and is well adjusted to it, and you would like to introduce some bones, you can consider feeding whole chicken and turkey parts, such as backs and necks, or halved or whole Cornish game hens, from time to time. However, excess bone, as well as bone fragments, can cause constipation and even intestinal impaction (which may involve an emergency surgery that your vet does not love doing), so don't overdo it!

Common sense always needs to be exercised, because in the long run, how well bones fit into your Paleo Dog plan all depends on the size, age, and health of your dog. When you are well into your transition (which may be months or even years from that last meal of kibble), use the combination of chunky muscle and organ meat as described in the Basic Recipe in Chapter 8, including the recommended supplements. Getting some food into your dog's gut before she gnaws on a bone provides a cushion in her stomach before the bones go down; tendons and fascia in the meat can wrap and protect the bones as they pass through the intestines. Remember, wild Paleo Dogs eat the bones last when there is already food in their stomachs.

When your dog is healthy enough to transition to bones that aren't incorporated directly into the food, those bones must be:

- **Fresh** (bones exposed to the air will harden more quickly than you might imagine; discard all bones at the end of the day)
- **Raw** (cooked bones will splinter and can easily crack teeth; dried-out raw bones can, too)
- **Appropriately sized** (small enough for the dog to chew but not small enough to choke)
- **Cancellous or spongy,** such as knucklebones, necks, and vertebrae (don't give cortical bones, the long straight bones such as ribs and leg bones)
- **Supervised** (many a dog has choked on a piece of bone, or broken a tooth, or gotten a bone stuck in the mouth or

throat; you need to be close by in case a problem occurs)

Large dogs really relish a raw, meaty knucklebone to gnaw on after a good meal. Raw bones are a true canine dessert and help prevent tartar. But they shouldn't be on the menu until you feel you are ready to go all-out Paleo! It is always best to err on the side of caution. These tips are essential in making an easy transition to the Paleo plan and will truly benefit your dog.

We like to prepare raw meat and then offer raw bones for dessert (as mentioned before, eating bones on a full stomach helps provide a bit of a cushion and protect the stomach). Simply let the raw meat and/or raw meaty bones defrost in diluted grapefruit seed extract solution (see the recipe in Chapter 8) in the refrigerator in a covered glass bowl. Or let fresh raw bones marinate in this solution to kill surface bacteria.

Raw bones are an essential part of being a Paleo Dog. Dental disease is the number one problem veterinarians see in dogs; it is usually established before age 3. Bones of any kind are, admittedly, controversial. But observing a few simple steps will enable you to feed bones safely.

Remember: Only raw is raw. Bones that

are smoked, flavored, boiled, baked, or processed in any way are not raw. Many of the problems vets see in dogs who eat bones come from a failure to observe this rule.

The adult deer or elk carcass a wolf pack leaves behind has only a head, a spine, ribs, legs, and hooves, plus some stomach and intestinal contents. The cartilage on the ends of bones is consumed. Young or small prey are completely consumed. Smaller scavengers pick off everything else that's edible, and small herbivorous animals like porcupines and rodents gnaw the edges of the bones for calcium.

Fresh raw bones will give your dog hours of chomping pleasure and entertainment, and will naturally remove surface plaque and stimulate the gums and other supporting structures for a healthy mouth.

For large dogs, fresh raw knucklebones or beef or bison oxtails (from grass-fed livestock, if possible) are a wonderful choice, as are turkey necks. For small dogs, whole or cut chicken necks are the bones of choice. Select poultry bones from free-range, pasture-raised sources when you can. For very small dogs and puppies, smash chicken necks with a meat mallet.

A dog not given bones still needs to satisfy his need to chew and gnaw on something satisfying. But left to his own devices, the items he chooses may be harmful, expensive, inconvenient, or irreplaceable, like the TV remote or Italian leather shoes!

ACID-ALKALINE BALANCE

Many people today are promoting an alkaline or an alkalinizing diet. This refers to pH, which is simply a measurement of how acidic or alkaline (basic) a liquid is. However, the pH of the diet primarily affects the pH of the urine, not the blood. A high-protein diet produces an acidic urine pH, while herbivores produce very alkaline urine on their diet of plants. Blood pH, however, is always maintained around 7.4 (7.35 to 7.45), regardless of the diet or pH of the drinking water. Any variation beyond those tight limits results in serious illness or death. Excess acid and base molecules are primarily regulated by the respiratory and urinary systems. Urine pH is not at all a reflection of the pH of the blood. Trying to regulate your dog's whole-body pH through alkaline food or water is misguided at best. Just feed your dog what dogs have been eating for thousands of years, provide good fresh drinking water, and leave the acid-base balance to Nature.

THE IMPORTANCE OF
PURE DRINKING WATER

Not all water is created equal. The kind of water your dog drinks can have a major impact on her health. Any water source can be filtered to make it healthier for your dog. The basic categories of water are municipal tap water, well water, distilled water, and spring water. We'll talk about each in turn.

Tap water. The quality of tap water varies tremendously from one municipality to another. Municipal water generally contains chlorine, fluoride, and harmful contaminants such as bacteria, arsenic, toxic pesticide residues, heavy metals, and even rocket fuel. Fluoride in particular is a suspect in certain types of kidney and liver damage, as well as hypothyroidism. Some cities' water tastes bad, but taste is not a reliable indicator of what's really in there.

If you must use tap water, it should be filtered so your dog can safely drink it. Even a simple countertop filter will remove chlorine, lead, arsenic, bacteria, and some chemicals. Faucet-mount or canister filters are a step up; under-sink or whole-house filters are best. You'll find many brands and a huge variation in price, but in general, you get what you pay for. Reverse-osmosis filtered water should have trace minerals added.

Well water. Well water may be pure and healthful, or it may be full of pathogenic organisms, agricultural runoff, heavy metals, and other contaminants. The only way to be sure is to have the water tested. Again, filtration may be the best option if your water is from a well.

Distilled water. Distilled water has been purified so that it does not contain any particles at all. While purity may sound good, you should not use distilled water for daily drinking. Distilled water contains zero solutes, so when it enters the intestines, diffusion will actually pull solutes out of the body. Drinking only distilled water can ultimately cause deficiencies in sodium, potassium, and important trace minerals. While distilled water can be valuable when used for a short-term process of detoxification, it's not safe for long-term consumption unless you add trace minerals to it (see Resources on page 537).

Spring water. If it's really from a natural spring and if the spring itself is good quality, spring water is the best choice for dogs — and the rest of the family, too! In general, avoid generic and grocery store brands because many of them test positive for bacteria and chemical contaminants, such as arsenic, chloroform, toluene, nitrates, and phthalates. Instead buy artesian spring water, which is purer because the layers of rock and clay around artesian aquifers provide protection from potential contamination.

You can provide the best food and great supplements for your dog, but if the water is poor quality, optimal health will remain out of reach. Pure, good-quality water is an essential ingredient of your dog's wellness program.

CHAPTER 8
PALEO DOG RECIPES

Now that you've learned the principles of the Paleo Dog Diet, it's time to get going! The following recipes are given for large batches of food (based on approximately 3 pounds of meat or organs). They can be divided into meal-size portions and frozen for up to 3 months.

Here are some general instructions:

- Buy whole cuts of meat if possible, and have your butcher grind it fresh, or grind it yourself at home. Any grocery store will do this for you. Never use nonorganic ground beef; the conventional beef industry's chronic lack of hygiene creates an unacceptably high level of bacterial contamination.
- All raw meat should be treated with 4 drops of grapefruit seed extract in 8 ounces of purified water before use.
- As much as possible, use organic

213

products, grass-fed meat, eggs from pastured hens, and raw dairy products.
- All liver, and preferably all organ meats, must be organic.
- Always follow safe meat-handling procedures.
- Dogs cannot digest raw fruits and vegetables; to get the maximum nutritional value from plant products, they must be "predigested" by cooking or pureeing.

Once your dog is fully transitioned to the Paleo Dog Diet, the daily meal plan should include at least two meals from the Complete Meals category. After at least 30 days on Complete Meal recipes, Fun Fare meals may be substituted for one Complete Meal up to three times per week as long as all indicated supplements are added. After that, you may substitute Fun Fare meals without supplements up to two times per week. Treats are just that — treats — and are designed to be used in moderation. All treats contribute calories to the diet, and they should be limited if your dog needs to lose weight.

The following recipe is the basic one Celeste has used and recommended successfully for thousands of pets for the past

20-plus years, and Jean has long recommended it for her clients and also uses it for her own pets. Your holistic veterinarian can help customize it for dogs with special needs.

Important: Please read through the basic recipe carefully before you begin to prepare your dog's first homemade meal. We know it may seem complicated, but after you make this recipe a few times, it will become so easy that you won't believe you waited so long to make your dog's food at home. And making food in your own kitchen, with your own hands, is how you add love as an essential ingredient! Your dog will enjoy waiting to savor this labor of love.

Use common sense when feeding your dog a homemade raw-meat diet. For example, some dogs enjoy certain vegetables, while others resist them. You'll need to experiment to see what works best.

THE PALEO DOG DIET
BASIC RECIPE

2 pounds organic, 100% grass-fed or pasture-raised raw diced beef or coarse-ground organic, cage-free poultry, up to 20 to 25 percent fat (Do not use pork or fish; limit ground lamb because of its high fat content.) Also try venison, elk, bison,

215

ostrich, quail, and other poultry, and alternate and/or combine meats for variety. (All meat should be frozen for 72 hours to kill parasitic cysts prior to feeding.)

8 ounces purified water combined with 4 drops of 0grapefruit seed extract liquid concentrate

1/2 pound raw minced or diced organic organ meat, such as liver (organic only), kidney, heart, and gizzard (turkey, chicken, beef, or lamb)

4 level tablespoons Celestial Pets VitaMineral Plus supplement for a homemade raw-meat diet (or similar alternative; use manufacturer's recommended amount)

Fats and fatty acids: 1 tin (4 ounces) sardines in extra virgin olive oil or Celestial Pets Essential Fatty Acid Oil; and a marine-source omega-3 supplement such as Moxxor (see Resources)

2 drops liquid garlic extract such as Kyolic Aged Garlic Extract (Since too much garlic can cause serious health consequences, do not oversupplement, and never use raw garlic.)

1/4 to 1/2 teaspoon Celestial Pets Enzyme Supplement or other digestive enzymes

Pinch of Himalayan or Celtic sea salt

500 milligrams taurine (powder or capsule)

for breeds predisposed to taurine deficiency related heart disease

Up to 16 ounces steamed, pureed non-starchy vegetables, such as organic zucchini or yams; or organic canned pumpkin; or organic baby food vegetables such as sweet potatoes or yams, carrots, or winter squash (Don't use corn or potatoes.)

1. For small mouths, you can have your butcher grind poultry backs and necks — or even a whole chicken. Be sure the butcher runs them through the grinder at least three times. You can also purchase your own meat grinder and grind your own meats and poultry. Or, use a mallet to crush whole chicken necks for smaller dogs. Feed whole bones only on a full stomach. (See Chapter 7 for more on feeding raw bones.)

2. Treat the meat/poultry with the purified water–grapefruit seed extract (GSE) liquid concentrate. Note: *Never* use GSE straight (internally or externally); it will cause serious chemical burns. It must always be properly diluted. To treat ground meat, place the meat in a bowl and pour the diluted GSE over it in small amounts, blending it into the meat as you go. Use

only enough of this solution as necessary to make the food the consistency of thick chili. For whole cuts, meat chunks, and necks, defrost them in this solution in the refrigerator.

3. Cut organs and large pieces of meat into bite-size chunks according to your dog's size. Liver (organic only) can be cut partially frozen. Meat, organs, and chicken necks can marinate in the GSE solution to kill surface bacteria while defrosting.

4. In a large bowl, mix all ingredients together. Serve.

(See "Nutritional Supplements" in Resources for suppliers of the supplements mentioned in this recipe.)

Refrigerate oils and Kyolic garlic after opening.

Starting Puppies on the Basic Paleo Dog Recipe

There are two nutritional standards for manufactured pet food — growth (puppy, pregnancy, nursing) and adult. All other life stages and "special needs" foods like individual breeds and lifestyles are essentially made up; they're mainly marketing tools.

Wild canines, once they start eating solid food, consume the same diet their entire lives. As we've seen, despite claims from veterinarians and the pet food and pharmaceutical industries that dogs are living longer, dogs' current life expectancy is very similar to that of the potential life span of their wild counterparts.[1]

Puppies may be introduced to small amounts of solid food at 5 weeks old, while they are still nursing. Increase the amounts as the puppy grows, until by 12 weeks they are receiving about 2 to 3 percent of their expected adult body weight per day, divided into at least three or four meals.

If your puppy is still eating some or all commercial pet food, especially dry kibble, at the time of spaying or neutering, reduce the amount fed by 20 to 30 percent per day. (If you're already feeding a raw diet, this may not be necessary.) A dog's metabolic requirements decrease as soon as the reproductive organs are removed, and a high-carb dry food diet is a very concentrated source of calories. If your puppy has already been spayed or neutered at the time of adoption, start with 2 percent of his or her projected adult weight, and adjust as needed.

At maturity (after 1 year of age for most dogs; a month or two later for giant breeds), most dogs can be fed twice a day. Feeding only one meal per day is a risk factor for bloat. Dogs and puppies reach their proper weight on the Paleo Dog Diet when fed according to their needs.

Overfeeding and over-supplementation (especially with calcium) can cause serious health problems like developmental bone disease, including hypertrophic osteodystrophy and osteochondrosis, especially in large and giant breed dogs.[2] It is crucial not to allow large and giant breed puppies to become overweight.

Amount to Feed
Pet food companies have done their best to train us to feed our dogs the same amount of the same food every day. But this doesn't even make sense when you think about how Paleo Dogs evolved. They ate what they could get, when they could get it. Of course, we have much better control over how much food our dogs can access, but there is no "one size fits all" rule for determining exactly how much to feed any individual dog on any particular day.

In general, start adult dogs on the Paleo Dog Diet by offering approximately 2 to 3 percent of their ideal body weight in food per day, split into at least 2 meals. Remove any food that is not eaten within 30 minutes, and feed less at the following meal. If your dog gobbles every morsel and still acts like he's starving, wait a half hour and give a little more.

Just like you don't eat the same amount or the same thing every day, your dog's appetite will fluctuate based on weather, season, activity level, and many other factors. If you both got a lot of exercise in the morning, you'll both be hungrier that night — so feed a little more at mealtime, or use a Fun Fare or Treat recipe as an evening snack.

Puppies will eat about twice as much food per pound as an adult dog, but food should be split into multiple small feedings to avoid vomiting from an overfilled stomach. As they grow, the actual amount eaten per pound of body weight naturally diminishes until they reach their full adult weight.

Large breed puppies should not receive more than 3 percent of their expected adult weight in food per day; excess calories may cause skeletal abnormalities. Do not add extra calcium to a large breed puppy's meals.

Pregnant or lactating females have higher nutritional requirements, and they will also be hungrier! Use common sense, pay attention, and feed her according to her demands.

You can make large batches and freeze in serving sizes appropriate for your dog(s).

We recommend certain products by name because all products marketed today are not equal (see Resources on page 529).

Raw Food Recipe Tips

Please check with your holistic practitioner before changing your dog's diet, as any change can be stressful.

If organ meat is difficult to obtain, include a variety of gland and organ concentrates (see Resources). *Note:* Celestial Pets VitaMineral Plus contains glandular and organ powder, so concentrates are not needed when using this product.

Use a supplement designed for a homemade meat-based diet, such as the Celestial Pets supplements, which were specifically designed by a veterinarian for the Basic Paleo Dog Recipe. The supplement(s) you choose should include correct proportions of bone meal, super greens, and gland and organ powder to balance the recipe properly.

Always defrost meat in the refrigerator,

---

not a counter, sink, or bowl of water.

Use only glass or ceramic (lead-free glazed) bowls. Plastic and stainless steel are microscopically porous and impossible to sterilize, and stainless steel can hold a charge and give your dog's nose a shock of static electricity.

Safe handling of raw meat is imperative. Wash hands, dishes, and utensils in hot, soapy water. Clean surfaces with environmentally safe cleaning products, such as a solution of 1 drop of grapefruit seed extract per ounce (30 milliliters) of water.

Leave food down for approximately 30 minutes. If it's too warm in the dog's eating area, or if flies become a problem, shorten the time. Unrefrigerated meat spoils quickly.

Increase portions or feed more small meals if your dog gobbles it all up and wants more; amounts can vary from meal to meal. But do not overfeed. A good guideline is to feed 2 to 3 percent of your adult dog's ideal weight. If your dog gains or loses too much weight, adjust feeding amounts.

Keep food in the refrigerator for no more than 3 days; beyond that, spoilage is likely. Store the food in glass bowls with tight lids.

If stools are too hard or dry or your dog strains to pass them, add up to 3 teaspoons of ground chia or flax-seeds per pound of meat.

Most important, prepare and serve with love!

HOMEMADE HEALING

Clear Day Chicken Broth (page 246)

Restoration Liver Puree (page 247)

COMPLETE MEALS

Please understand that we cannot guarantee that these recipes are "100 percent complete and balanced" according to the standards set by the AAFCO, standards which are imperfect, as we have noted, but they are the only game in town. For one thing, plants and animals grown in different places at different times vary widely in their precise nutritional content. Pet food manufacturers add large overdoses of vitamins and minerals to compensate for deficiencies in their ingredients, as well as for nutrient loss during processing and storage. However, our philosophy differs from the pet food companies' in that we don't think each and every meal needs to be a nutritionally complete, self-contained package. Rather, we believe that by feeding a variety of fresh, wholesome meats and vegetables, basic supplements, and healthy treats, the dog's diet will be balanced over time. This is exactly how humans have managed to survive our first 300,000 years; it's how we all grew up, and how we continue to live every day. It's how wild canids have always lived; they don't select one type of prey to the exclusion of all others — they eat what they can get. And we trust that, between Mother Nature and your own common sense, your dog will thrive, too!

Silky Skin and Coat Formula

For dogs with skin conditions and allergies.

2 pounds ground organic ostrich (or other nonallergic meat)

1/2 pound organic chicken liver, chopped

1 can (16 ounces) organic yams or 1 pound fresh garnet yams, baked or steamed

1 tablespoon organic coconut oil

2 tablespoons organic ground chia seeds or flaxseed meal

2 level tablespoons Celestial Pets VitaMineral Plus supplement for a homemade raw-meat diet (or similar alternative; use manufacturer's recommended amount)

Fats and fatty acids: 1 can (approx. 4 ounces) sardines in extra virgin olive oil or Celestial Pets Essential Fatty Acid Oil; and a marine-source omega-3 supplement such as Moxxor (see Resources)

1 drop liquid garlic extract such as Kyolic Aged Garlic Extract (Since too much garlic can cause serious health consequences, do not oversupplement, and never use raw garlic.)

1/8 to 1/4 teaspoon Celestial Pets Enzyme Supplement or other digestive enzymes

Pinch of Himalayan or Celtic sea salt

In a large bowl, mix all ingredients together. Serve.

Flexible Joint Formula

For large and older dogs to maintain or improve joint function.

2 pounds organic chicken or turkey with bone (ground fresh by the butcher or at home)

1/2 cup steamed pureed organic veggies (kale, chard, broccoli, spinach, brussels sprouts, carrots)

2 level tablespoons Celestial Pets VitaMineral Plus supplement for a homemade raw-meat diet (or similar alternative; use manufacturer's recommended amount)

Fats and fatty acids: 1 can (approx. 4 ounces) sardines in extra virgin olive oil or Celestial Pets Essential Fatty Acid Oil; and a marine-source omega-3 supplement such as Moxxor (see Resources)

1 drop liquid garlic extract such as Kyolic Aged Garlic Extract (Since too much garlic can cause serious health consequences, do not oversupplement, and never use raw garlic.)

1/8 to 1/4 teaspoon Celestial Pets Enzyme Supplement or other digestive enzymes

Pinch of Himalayan or Celtic sea salt

1,500 milligrams glucosamine sulfate
1,000 milligrams collagen powder
500 milligrams hyaluronic acid
500 milligrams Yucca schidigera root powder

In a large bowl, mix all ingredients together. Serve.

Brain Food Formula
For working or older dogs to maintain or improve cognitive function.

2 pounds ground organic, 100% grass-fed or pasture-raised red meat (lean beef, bison, elk, venison)
1/2 pound organic beets, baked or steamed and pureed
1/2 cup organic blueberries
1 tablespoon organic coconut oil
2 tablespoons organic ground chia seeds
2 level tablespoons Celestial Pets VitaMineral Plus supplement for a homemade raw-meat diet (or similar alternative; use manufacturer's recommended amount)
Fats and fatty acids: 1 can (approx. 4 ounces) sardines in extra virgin olive oil or Celestial Pets Essential Fatty Acids Oil; and a marine-source omega-3 supplement such as Moxxor (see Resources)

231

1 drop liquid garlic extract such as Kyolic Aged Garlic Extract (Since too much garlic can cause serious health consequences, do not oversupplement, and never use raw garlic.)

1/8 to 1/4 teaspoon Celestial Pets Enzyme Supplement or other digestive enzymes

Pinch of Himalayan or Celtic sea salt

In a large bowl, mix all ingredients together. Serve.

Power Meat Loaf

For hardworking dogs who need high-energy sustenance.

1 pound ground organic chicken thighs

1 pound ground organic, 100% grass-fed New Zealand lamb

1 can (13.2 ounces) green tripe

8 ounces ground organic, 100% grass-fed or pasture-raised organ meat, such as heart, gizzard, kidney, liver, spleen (melts), etc.

3 tablespoons plain organic yogurt or 2 organic egg yolks

1 tablespoon chopped parsley, dulse flakes, or kelp powder

3 tablespoons chopped organic black olives

2 tablespoons organic ground chia seeds or

flaxseed meal

2 level tablespoons Celestial Pets VitaMineral Plus supplement for a homemade raw-meat diet (or similar alternative; use manufacturer's recommended amount)

Fats and fatty acids: 1 can (approx. 4 ounces) sardines in extra virgin olive oil or Celestial Pets Essential Fatty Acids Oil; and a marine-source omega-3 supplement such as Moxxor (see Resources)

1 drop liquid garlic extract such as Kyolic Aged Garlic Extract (Since too much garlic can cause serious health consequences, do not oversupplement, and never use raw garlic.)

1/8 to 1/4 teaspoon Celestial Pets Enzyme Supplement or other digestive enzymes

Pinch of Himalayan or Celtic sea salt

1 cup organic whey powder (optional)

1 cup organic steamed pureed carrots or sweet potatoes (optional)

In a large bowl, mix all ingredients together. Serve.

Fun Fare

The following Fun Fare recipes do not replace the Basic Paleo Dog Diet, as they do not contain the full complement of recommended daily supplements. They are intended for occasional use only. If you wish to use any of these recipes as a balanced meal, simply add the supplements recommended in the Basic Paleo Dog Diet, which will provide the necessary nutrients for more frequent feeding.

Paleo Wraps

A portable meal or snack for dogs on the go.

2 pounds ground organic turkey
2 pounds minced organic beef heart
2 raw organic eggs (preferably pasture-raised)
1 tablespoon organic extra virgin olive oil
1 bunch organic romaine lettuce or 1 pack-

age nori (seaweed) sheets
1 can (approx. 4 ounces) sardines

1. In a large bowl, mix together the turkey, beef heart, eggs, and olive oil.

2. Spread the mixture on the romaine leaves or nori sheets, leaving about 1″ on one side without filling. Place a sardine on the filling at the edge of a leaf or sheet. Roll it up by hand or using a sushi mat so that the sardine is in the center. If using nori, moisten the bare edge to seal.

3. Slice the wraps to the desired size.

Chili-Less Chili
A blend of antioxidant herbs and spices boosts this meal's vitality.

3 pounds diced, organic, 100% grass-fed beef or bison
1 can (16 ounces) organic red kidney beans
1 can (16 ounces) organic stewed tomatoes
1 tablespoon fresh organic parsley, finely chopped
3 drops Kyolic Aged Garlic Extract
1 teaspoon dried oregano
1 teaspoon dried basil
1 teaspoon ground cumin

2 teaspoons ground turmeric
3 tablespoons organic extra virgin olive oil
Digestive enzymes
1 tablespoon chopped cilantro and/or a dollop of organic crème fraîche or sour cream for garnish (optional)

In a large bowl, mix all of the ingredients together and, if desired, serve over a raw chicken or turkey neck slice of the appropriate size, topped with cilantro and/or crème fraîche or sour cream.

Canine Curry
Packed with vitamins and antioxidants.

1/2 cup organic cream
1/2 cup plain (full-fat) organic Greek yogurt
1 teaspoon grated fresh ginger
1 tablespoon mild curry powder
2 drops Kyolic Aged Garlic Extract
Pinch of Himalayan or Celtic sea salt
1 cup cooked or canned organic lentils
8 ounces frozen or fresh raw organic green beans, chopped
2 large organic carrots, shredded
1 small can organic diced tomatoes
Low-salt, organic chicken broth
3 tablespoons butter (optional)
2 pounds organic chicken and/or 100%

grass-fed lamb, cubed

Chopped organic parsley, cilantro, slivered almonds, and/or dried goji berries for garnish (optional)

1. In a large pot, combine the cream, yogurt, ginger, curry powder, garlic, and salt. Mix in the lentils, green beans, carrots, and tomatoes. Add chicken broth and butter, if using, as needed for desired texture. Mix well and simmer to thicken.

2. Add the raw meat. Top with the herbs, almonds, and/or goji berries, if using.

Steak Shish Kebab

The Paleo way for your dog to share barbecue time with family and friends!

Marinade

1/2 cup organic, extra virgin olive oil

1/4 cup organic apple cider or balsamic vinegar

1/4 cup organic orange juice

Sprig of fresh organic rosemary

1 drop Kyolic Aged Garlic Extract

Pinch of Himalayan or Celtic sea salt

Kebabs

1 pound organic, 100% grass-fed or pasture-raised flank steak

1 pound organic, 100% grass-fed or pasture-raised beef heart

1/2 pound organic celery and/or carrots

Assorted organic vegetables (zucchini, yellow squash, broccoli, cauliflower, tomatoes)

Organic mushrooms (button, cremini, or portobello)

1. In a large bowl, mix all of the marinade ingredients together.

2. Cut the flank steak into sections and cut a slit in the middle of each piece. Slice the beef heart into cross-sections (so the open chambers are in the middle).

3. Marinate the steak and heart slices for 15 minutes.

4. While the meat is marinating, make edible "skewers" from the celery ribs and/or carrots by slicing them lengthwise. Slice the vegetables and mushrooms, if large.

5. Drain and discard the marinade and rosemary sprig. Alternately skewer the veggie

slices, flank steak, mushrooms, and beef heart slices on a celery or carrot skewer.

6. Serve raw.

Note: You can easily share the same meal as your dog! Follow these preparations except use wooden skewers instead of veggie sticks (soak skewers in salted water for 15 minutes before cooking to prevent them from catching fire) and grill the kebabs to your desired doneness.

Bully Burgers
Good for brains as well as brawn!

2 pounds fresh 85% lean ground organic, 100% grass-fed beef or bison
2 cups finely chopped fresh organic spinach
2 cups chopped fresh organic tomatoes
1 cup crumbled organic feta cheese or cubed organic mozzarella, Swiss, or Cheddar cheese
2 tablespoons omega-3 oil (Celestial Pets; or anchovy, sardine, or herring oil)
2 drops Kyolic Aged Garlic Extract
1/4 teaspoon Himalayan or Celtic sea salt

1. In a large bowl, mix all of the ingredients together.

2. Form into burger patties.

3. Serve raw.

Slippery Sliders

2 pounds fresh 90% lean ground organic, 100% grass-fed beef or bison
4 drops Kyolic Aged Garlic Extract

1. In a large bowl, combine the meat and garlic drops.

2. Form into small patties.

3. Serve on sliced Cheesy Biscuits (page 244) or Paleo Scones (page 242).

Quadriped Quiche

4 eggs, beaten
1 tablespoon cream
1/2 cup cubed organic meat (any type)
1/2 cup shredded organic vegetables (tomatoes, mushrooms, zucchini, squash)
2 ounces shredded organic white or yellow cheese

1. Preheat the oven to 450°F.

2. In a glass 9″ pie plate, combine all of the ingredients and stir well.

3. Bake for 15 minutes. Reduce the heat to 375°F and bake for 25 minutes.

4. Remove from the oven and allow the quiche to set for 5 minutes.

5. Allow to cool before serving.

TREATS

These treat recipes contain gluten-free, low-carb flour to provide texture.

Paleo Scones
3 1/2 cups organic quinoa flour
1 cup organic buttermilk
1 cup shredded organic mozzarella cheese, divided
4 tablespoons organic butter, melted
2 teaspoons aluminum-free baking soda
1 teaspoon Himalayan or Celtic sea salt

1. Preheat the oven to 350°F.

2. In a large bowl, mix the flour and the buttermilk to form a thick dough.

3. Blend in 3/4 cup of the cheese, the butter, baking soda, and salt.

4. On a work surface, knead and flatten the

dough three times. Then flatten or roll out until 3/4″ thick.

5. Score with a knife, cookie cutter, or pizza roller into the desired size and shape. Cut out and place on an ungreased baking sheet.

6. Top with the remaining 1/4 cup cheese.

7. Bake for 40 minutes, or until slightly brown.

Carrot Cookies

1 cup organic coconut oil
2 organic, pasture-raised eggs
1/2 cup organic unsulfured molasses
2 cups organic coconut flour
1 teaspoon ground cinnamon
1 teaspoon ground ginger
2 teaspoons aluminum-free baking powder
Pinch of Himalayan or Celtic sea salt
2 cups steamed, mashed carrots (or baked or steamed and mashed sweet potatoes)

1. Preheat the oven to 375°F. Grease a baking sheet or line a baking sheet with oiled parchment paper.

2. In a medium bowl, mix the coconut oil,

eggs, and molasses.

3. In a large bowl, combine the coconut flour, cinnamon, ginger, baking powder, and salt.

4. Gradually add the mashed carrots (or sweet potatoes) and the oil-egg mixture to the dry ingredients. Mix well to form a dough.

5. Drop by bite-size spoonfuls onto the baking sheet. Bake for 12 minutes, or until browned.

Cheesy Biscuits
4 organic, pasture-raised eggs
1/4 cup melted organic butter or coconut oil
1/4 teaspoon Himalayan or Celtic sea salt
1/3 cup organic coconut flour or quinoa flour
1/4 teaspoon aluminum-free baking powder
1 tablespoon ground organic chia seeds (Salba)
1 cup shredded organic medium or sharp Cheddar cheese

1. Preheat the oven to 400°F. Line a baking

sheet with parchment paper.

2. In a large bowl, blend together the eggs, butter or coconut oil, and salt.

3. Add the flour, baking powder, and chia seeds, and whisk the batter until there are no lumps.

4. Fold in the cheese.

5. Drop the batter by bite-size spoonfuls onto the baking sheet.

6. Bake for 15 minutes, or until a wooden pick inserted in the center comes out clean.

Homemade Healing

Clear Day Chicken Broth

Use this clear broth for tummy upsets such as vomiting or loose stool. If symptoms are severe or persist for more than 24 hours, seek veterinary care.

1 whole organic chicken
1 cup chopped organic celery
1 cup chopped organic carrots

1. In a large pot or slow cooker, combine all of the ingredients and cover with purified water.

2. Simmer (or cook in the slow cooker on low) until the chicken falls off the bone (usually several hours).

3. Strain the broth through a fine-mesh strainer or cheesecloth.

4. Reserve the cooked chicken; dice and mix with white rice for reintroducing solid food.

5. Discard the carrots and celery (or use for human consumption).

Restoration Liver Puree

For recovery from illness or surgery; ideal for dogs who have feeding tubes.

1 pound organic chicken liver or organic, 100% grass-fed beef liver

2 capsules Moxxor or other marine omega-3 oil (remove from capsule)

2 level tablespoons Celestial Pets VitaMineral Plus (or alternative vitamin-mineral blend; use manufacturer's recommended amount)

1/8 to 1/4 teaspoon Celestial Pets Enzyme Supplement or other digestive enzymes

Water or organic chicken broth as needed to attain the desired consistency

Optional: Raw organic whole cream (not ultra-pasteurized) or organic butter (do not use butter in a feeding tube)

1. Cut the liver into chunks. In a blender, combine the liver, omega-3 oil, supple-

ments, water or broth, and cream (if using).

2. Puree to the desired consistency.

3. Strain the mixture if using in a feeding tube.

CHAPTER 9
POTENTIAL PROBLEMS
AND SOLUTIONS

Okay, now that you're ready to get your dog on the road to optimal health, what could possibly go wrong? Well, there are a few issues that tend to occur when making radical diet and lifestyle changes, and it's important to be prepared for them. The following are frequently voiced issues and concerns, with plenty of information to help you understand and implement the Paleo Dog Program safely and effectively.

MY DOG SEEMS WORSE ON A RAW DIET

While we absolutely believe that the healthiest diet for a dog is the raw meat–based Paleo Dog Diet, there are always exceptions. That's why we recommend a gradual introduction of the diet. If your dog has always eaten processed dry food, it may take many months of careful persistence to achieve the goal of a Paleo Dog Diet. Some dogs may never get there; they may need to have their food cooked, or they may need extra carbohydrates. Some dogs do better with cooked grains; some without vegetables.

Your dog is like a black box — you simply cannot know about all the genetic and epigenetic heritage embedded in your dog's cells. What your dog's parents, grandparents, and even great-grandparents ate, what vaccinations they received, what medicines they took — these all have an effect on your dog today. What we are trying to do with the Paleo Dog Diet and Lifestyle is to raise your dog to the maximum healthiest level that can possibly be achieved, given the many factors at play that are not within our control. Obviously, we can't all take our dogs to an unspoiled environment and let them run like wolves, but we can at least begin to move them in that direction.

That being said, many holistic veterinarians still recommend a homemade raw diet along the Paleo Dog lines. But they also acknowledge — and caution — that every dog is unique, and not every dog is a suitable candidate for the full Paleo Dog Diet and Lifestyle. We cannot say this strongly enough: Please find a holistic vet to work with one-on-one to make sure your dog is making progress and to address any specific issues that may arise.

MY VET SAYS A
RAW DIET ISN'T SAFE

Most conventional vets who are against a raw diet have no real experience with it, and have not seen the science that supports it. We encourage you to read the following and to share it with your vet — we lay out the scientific case in favor of a homemade raw diet and then discuss the two primary objections that conventional veterinarians typically have against this diet: contamination of raw meat by pathogenic organisms and lack of nutritional balance.

As we've seen, dogs belong to the order Carnivora — the meat-eaters. A dog's teeth are pointy, sharp, and obviously made for puncturing, gripping, and ripping. These dental characteristics evolved some 63 million years ago and have not changed since then. Dogs' jaws are muscular and powerful; they're well suited to capturing and consuming prey animals of all sizes, but they cannot move side to side to chew. Dogs do not have large, flat molars for chewing, as do humans, deer, and pigs. Even bears' teeth are much better adapted to a diet that includes plant matter.

Canids have been eating the same thing

— prey animals — for at least 30 million years. As we learned in Chapter 2, although man and wolf have been co-existing — maybe closely — for millennia, the earliest date for domestication of the wolf (*Canis lupus*), which is also the origin of the dog (*Canis lupus familiaris*), is around 35,000 years ago; that's mere moments on an evolutionary scale. Dog and wolf DNA remain nearly identical today. Selective breeding has created hundreds of different-*looking* dogs, but changes in size and appearance, and even in temperament and behavior, aren't necessarily correlated to physiology.

Some experts argue that most humans are ill-equipped to digest current dietary staples like cereal grains (especially wheat and corn) because they were not part of our evolutionary history. Nevertheless, studies in humans show very little difference in the basic structure and function of the digestive system among racial groups — including those who still eat a primitive diet — even though the agricultural revolution occurred 10,000 years ago.

Dog biscuits were first created in the 1890s, but were not widely used. Canned food (mostly unsupplemented horsemeat) was popular in the 1930s. Today's commercial dry kibble gained widespread popularity in the United States only during World War II, when the supply of steel for cans was diverted from pets to weapons and machinery. Claims that dogs have somehow evolved within the last 75 years to be able to thrive on highly processed, grain-based pet food are completely bogus.

Most of our dogs' wild cousins still primarily eat prey, whose bodies consist of mostly water, protein, fat, and less than 10 percent (probably closer to 3 percent) carbohydrate, primarily as glycogen (the storage form of sugar in the liver) and whatever grasses, leaves, or other forage is in its digestive tract.

Despite their predatory heritage, members of the canine family are more accurately referred to as facultative or opportunistic omnivores; that is, they can survive on almost any type of food. During the summer, for example, wild foxes will eat a great deal of fruit and other vegetation. Feral dogs around the world subsist on whatever they can scrounge.

The modern dog is 99.8 percent wolf, but genetic changes have taken place that distinguish the two. New research on the dog's genome has discovered 122 of the genes that are in that 0.2 percent. In particular, dogs have from 4 to 30 copies of three specific genes that involve starch digestion and utilization, whereas wolves have only two. This implies that these genes provided an evolutionary advantage that arose during the process of domestication. Other changed genes involve the brain, nervous system, and adrenal glucocorticoids, which have to do with behavior and the stress response. Additionally, changes in genes involving reproductive capacity were also noted.[1]

Russian geneticist Dmitri Belyaev's farm fox experiment, discussed in Chapter 2, appears to support the manifestation of these changes. Besides obvious physical changes, tamer foxes also showed changes in reproduction; instead of breeding once a year in the spring, like wild and non-tame farm foxes do, tame foxes were able to breed at least two times per year. In addition, tamer foxes produce less adrenaline (the hormone that generates the fight-or-flight response), which may account for their reduced fear toward humans.[2]

Biologists are, for the most part, still stuck on Charles Darwin's dogma on evolution — believing that the only thing that changes genes is mutation, and that mutation is always a purely random event. But what seems to be more probable is something called adaptive mutation, in which the environment controls mutation.[3] As it turns out, signals from the environment can, through epigenetic mechanisms, control the expression of DNA. It is likely that the presence of increased dietary starch influenced which genes were used to the animal's advantage, and therefore which genes increased in frequency in the dog population. But no matter what the genes are or how many copies of them are present in the DNA, they are not really calling the shots on how the dog's digestive system functions.

So what is the significance of dogs having a variable number of extra genes for digesting starch? It depends on the dog's environment — and not only a particular dog's environment but also that of its parents and grandparents. This may explain why some dogs seem to do better on, or "need," starchier diets, and why others take to raw diets like ducks to water. Fortunately, because of the flexibility of epigenetics, it opens up the possibility that we can actually improve the genetic hand the dog was dealt — within that dog's lifetime.

Pet food manufacturers, of course, have gone to the opposite extreme. They have long taken advantage of dogs' nutritional flexibility to promote a wide variety of carbohydrate-filled foods that provide cheap nutrition (and astronomical profits!). They are no doubt thrilled to have hard science back up their preference for cheap starchy ingredients. But is this the best way to feed our dogs? In a word, no! Scientific research absolutely justifies a fresh food diet.

A study dubbed "Pottenger's Dogs," although it used only a few dogs, was conducted on growth and reproduction. (See Chapter 3 for the study "Pottenger's Cats.") Dogs received as a sole diet either raw, evaporated, or pasteurized milk supplemented with iron, copper, manganese, and cod liver oil. All dogs appeared healthy for 3 years on each regimen. However, reproduction — which places significant stress on the female body — was normal only in dogs fed the raw milk with cod liver oil. Muscle dystrophy and hemorrhage were observed in pups born to the dog fed pasteurized milk; those signs were even worse in the pups of the dog fed evaporated milk. Vitamin E supplementation prevented muscle dystrophy; vitamin K deficiency may have contributed to the hemorrhages.[4]

The effects of cooking vary, depending on the food. Vegetables and grains are generally made more digestible, but some vitamins are destroyed.[5] Cooking denatures proteins in meat but doesn't much change its nutritional value. In fact, because cooking evaporates about 10 percent of the moisture in meat, cooked meat's nutrient levels are, if anything, a little higher than those of raw meat.[6] However, what cooking does do to meat is reduce its nutritive value; in other words, the dog cannot absorb the same nutrition from cooked meat as it can from raw.[7] Dry food universally incorporates rendered meat and by-products; rendering is a process of boiling the raw ingredients, usually for hours. The same holds true for by-products when they're processed into kibble. But fresh and raw ingredients are 5 to 10 percent more nutritious than the same ingredients when rendered.[8]

This should come as no surprise to pet food makers. Research done in the 1930s showed that raw meat has a higher biological value than cooked or processed meat, and the differences are more pronounced the longer the meat is cooked.[9] Pet food makers know very well how processing, packaging, and storage affects each dog food ingredient, so they typically add 300 to 400 percent extra vitamins and other nutrients that may be diminished by those factors.[10] They also know how dogs digest and utilize those ingredients, and they

257

compensate for this as well. But the thing most pet food companies know the most about is palatability: how to get dogs to eat food that they would never encounter in nature.

CONTAMINATION

It's reasonable to assume that all meat in the United States is contaminated with bacteria, including *Salmonella* and *Campylobacter*, and other pathogenic organisms such as *Toxoplasma.* Some meats are worse than others, and we specifically recommend *against* feeding raw pork, fish, or non-organic ground beef because of the unacceptably high risk of parasitic and bacterial contamination. (See Appendix B on page 449 for a discussion of food-borne diseases.) We believe that following the Paleo Dog Diet does not present a risk to dogs or humans due to pathogenic organisms in meat, because:

- Dogs themselves are relatively resistant to meat-borne organisms, thanks to their strong stomach acid and relatively rapid gastrointestinal transit time.[11] This has been amply demonstrated by the fact that, despite dozens of recalls of many tons of processed dog food and treats because of bacterial contamination (particularly *Salmonella*), very few dogs have ever become sick from eating contaminated dry diets. Multiple studies of raw diets have found bacteria in the meat being fed; yet, no illnesses were reported in the dogs eating the food. Moreover, a significant percent of dogs are already carriers of one or more common pathogens.[12] Up to 36 percent of normal dogs (the vast majority of whom eat commercial dry dog food) are positive for *Salmonella.*[13] In fact, 52 percent of healthy dogs in one survey were carriers of pathogenic bacteria, including *Staph, Strep, Bacillus, E. coli,* and *Salmonella,* among others.[14]

- In the Paleo Dog Diet, we recommend treating all raw meat with an antimicrobial solution of diluted grapefruit seed extract (GSE).
- We encourage "newbies" to cook the meat, until they and/or their dogs become accustomed to the Paleo Dog method of feeding.
- Providing digestive enzymes and probiotics with meals helps to both break down pathogens and support normal

gastrointestinal flora, established populations of which naturally outcompete potentially invasive bacteria.[15]

- As far as zoonotic (animal-to-human disease transmission) risk, the Paleo Dog Diet specifically instructs that safe meat handling procedures should be followed at all times. Moreover, pets are not a significant source of zoonotic disease.[16]

LACK OF NUTRITIONAL BALANCE

A well-known phenomenon plaguing homemade diets is called diet drift. This is when clients start with a balanced recipe, but over time, they run out of this ingredient or forget about that one, and the diet becomes unbalanced. We acknowledge this problem, and we caution against it. Because we strongly encourage people to work with their veterinarian in implementing the Paleo Dog Program, and to take things one small step at a time, we sincerely hope that it can be followed correctly. However, we cannot guarantee that no one will ever make a mistake.

It's not easy to formulate a commercial pet food, either; to get all the nutrients right, it takes a $5,000 computer program, and many formulators also possess board certification from the American College of Veterinary Nutrition. There are fewer than 80 such individuals in the United States; many of them are directly employed by large pet food companies, and the bulk of the rest are in academia. The few independent nutritionists who are willing to formulate a complete pet diet are in high demand. It's exceedingly complicated, even though pet foods are required to provide only 36 individual nutrients.[17] Changing just one thing has a cascade of effects on every other ingredient.

Making homemade dog food is actually easier and results in a more nutritious food. Among the many available resources are the USDA Nutrient Database[18] and the USDA National Agricultural Library.[19] As opposed to the 36 required nutrients of the AAFCO Nutrient Profiles, the USDA database shows that ground turkey alone contains more than 90 nutrients.

The most common shortcoming of home-made diets is the calcium content. Many diets contain too much or too little of this vital mineral. We have seen diets that recommend that the food contain 10 percent calcium and others that fail to include any source of calcium at all. We have thoroughly studied this issue and are confident that the

Paleo Dog Diet contains an appropriate amount of calcium (about 1 percent of the diet) when fed as directed, using the Celestial Pets VitaMineral Plus supplement (which was formulated by a veterinarian for this purpose and has been fed successfully to many generations of show and breeding dogs) or an equivalent product.

In the Paleo Dog Diet, we also strongly recommend using grass-fed meat and pasture-raised poultry and eggs. Numerous studies have shown the superiority of these products over their conventionally raised counterparts. For example, 100 percent grass-fed/grass-finished beef contains an excellent array of fatty acids, while corn-finished beef has almost no omega-3s at all.[20]

A 2001 review of raw diets found that "all the [raw] diets tested had nutrient deficiencies or excesses that could cause serious health problems when used in a long-term feeding program."[21] Unfortunately, this was a badly flawed study that failed to truthfully report all of the results obtained. Two commercially prepared and three homemade diets were included in the study. The authors botched the analysis of the two commercial diets so badly that they had to publish a correction. For the homemade diets, the authors admit that "exact recipes of the diets were not provided to us." Even though the samples were assumed to be representative of the diets published by raw proponents, nobody checked to see whether those diets were actually being prepared according to those protocols — and clearly, they were not. For example, the article mentions that all of the homemade diets contained "entire breasts or legs of chickens." However, neither of those items are included in any of the three diet programs.

Moreover, diet samples were not collected in a reproducible manner. For example, the person who provided the authors with a sample based on Kymythy Schultze's *Ultimate Diet* told Schultze herself that, for 2 weeks, every time he fed the dog, he would throw a little bit of whatever he was feeding into a bag in the freezer. If he fed the dog a banana, he put a chunk of banana in the bag; and if he fed 2 pounds of meat, he added a little bit of meat. Any analysis of this mash-up was doomed to be hopelessly inaccurate.[22] Nevertheless, the authors drew several completely unwarranted conclusions from their incredibly sloppy research. Veterinarians still point to this study as if it were definitive, when it is as far away from "definitive" as it could possibly get.

If one lesson can be drawn from this terrible research, it is that people don't always follow directions. While we have provided instructions for the Paleo Dog Diet, there is no way to enforce how you choose to make the food and what specific ingredients you use. The good news is that it isn't necessary to have every meal be "perfect," just as you can't ensure perfection in your own diet. If you follow the guidelines, include the recommended supplements, and utilize a variety of meats and vegetables, your dogs' nutritional needs will, over time, be fulfilled.

MY VET SAYS RAW BONES ARE NOT SAFE

Another concern expressed by veterinarians is the risk associated with feeding raw bones. Raw bones can and do splinter, and they can cause impactions, perforations, and tooth fractures.

However, we are very specific about what bones to feed and how to feed them. If you follow the instructions in Chapter 7 carefully, the risk is vanishingly small.

The benefit of eating raw bones, in our opinion, outweighs any negative. There is much support in veterinary literature for the benefits of raw bones.

Animals need more "hassle factor" per

mouthful of nutrients. The literature contains hundreds of references to the food habits of feral carnivores and, therefore, the appropriate menu is readily available. Convenient prepared diets, those without sufficient "hassle factor," are ruining the mouths and compromising the health of our animals. Carnivores, in their natural habitat, eat rabbits, mice, rodents, birds, etc., in toto (i.e., connective tissues, viscera, organs). . . . The masticatory apparatus of carnivores was designed to be used, and used aggressively and ferociously. If the animals don't use their dentition and masticatory apparatus, they will in time lose it. The systemic health of any individual animal will not be adequately maintained with the loss of the primary entry mechanism to the digestive system."[23]

A 1-month study on Beagles found that the dogs' dental health was much improved when they were given half an oxtail once a week.[24] Another researcher concluded, "There is reasonable evidence that . . . foods requiring vigorous prehension and mastication are preferable for dogs and cats."[25] Raw bones and tissues provide this essential resistance.

Sir J. Frank Colyer, a pioneer in dental health, reported that the natural diets of wild canids and felids had a plaque-retardant effect, and that wild canids and felids did not have the generalized form of periodontal disease seen in domesticated pets.[26] Colyer's principles, including "[dental] disease is caused by an alteration in the character of the diet of the animal either of a physical or chemical nature — in other words, by a departure from natural diet and conditions," were fundamental in the 1982 founding of the Colyer Institute, which is dedicated to preserving dental health in exotic animals.

Another veterinary textbook author observed, "If dogs are injudiciously fed, receiving mostly soft food instead of that requiring tearing and chewing, the teeth become practically functionless, the gums become soft, and micro-organisms remain in contact therewith without disturbance, and eventually set up a gingivitis. The infection extends from the gum to the periodontal membrane, and thence to the surrounding bone, giving rise to a varying degree of toxaemia, manifested by different forms of constitutional disturbance."[27]

Finally, according to another textbook, "When animals feed in the wild they rarely develop a serious level of periodontal disease unless they are debilitated in some other way. By feeding animals unnatural foods we encourage plaque buildup and the development of periodontal disease."[28]

Somehow, in the years since the introduction of commercial dog food, the wisdom of generations has been lost. Periodontal disease is almost universal in today's dogs, who suffer under the influence of high profitability for pet food companies and the veterinarians who care for our dogs' diseased mouths.

DIARRHEA OR OTHER DIGESTIVE UPSET

Many dogs will have a change in stool color or consistency, from drier or chalky-looking to diarrhea, with a change of diet. (Any stool that is softer or more liquid than normal is medically considered to be diarrhea.) As long as the dog is still eating well and acting fine, mild diarrhea is normal, even if it persists for a few days or even a week or two. However, *if* your dog has *any* additional symptoms, such as lethargy, poor appetite, or persistent vomiting, stop the new food and contact your veterinarian. There may be something else going on!

Here are some ways to prevent or resolve

diarrhea due to diet change.

- Make the switch very slowly or decrease the amount of new food being fed and go back to a larger proportion of the old food.
- For 24 hours, feed only Clear Day Chicken Broth (see page 246).
- Temporarily (for up to 2 weeks) switch to plain boiled chicken with a small amount of canned pumpkin, cooked organic rice, or rice baby cereal. Add digestive enzymes but no other supplements. Use this as the basis for your switch to raw, instead of going back to the previous diet.
- Add extra digestive enzymes and probiotics to the basic recipe. Enzymes should be plant- or fungal-based and include protease, lipase, amylase, and cellulase. (See Resources on page 529 for suggestions.)
- Add marshmallow root or slippery elm bark powder to the food, or give a capsule or two to your dog up to 30 minutes before meals. These plants contain mucilage, which soothes and protects the intestinal lining, draws out impurities, and promotes healing. (See Chapter 11.)

VOMITING/REGURGITATION

If your dog is vomiting the new diet, he may be eating too fast. Try feeding meals in four to six small portions every 20 to 30 minutes, or use a specially made "slow-down" food bowl containing obstacles to prevent the gulping of food. (However, these bowls are usually plastic, so use them only as long as is needed to improve your dog's eating habits.)

Regurgitation is different from vomiting; it is a passive process (no retching or abdominal effort involved) in which the food slides back out of the mouth in the tubular shape of the esophagus. This may indicate a blockage in the upper gastrointestinal tract, and your dog should be evaluated by a veterinarian.

MUSCLE SORENESS

If your dog seems stiff or sore after unusually vigorous exercise, try some massage (see page 331). Additionally, the homeopathic remedy Arnica or the homotoxicology remedies Traumeel and Rendimax are good to have on hand for those particularly achy days.

You may wish to consult a holistic veterinarian to learn specific acupressure points and range-of-motion techniques you can use at home, especially for older or over-weight dogs who may have a harder time starting an exercise program.

DETOXIFICATION

A cornerstone of holistic medicine is the emphasis on symptoms being the immune system's way of calling for help. Absorption and accumulation of toxins in various tissues force the immune system to work harder to protect the body and keep it functioning normally. Eventually the immune system becomes overwhelmed, and various problems and symptoms develop that cause us to seek medical or veterinary treatment. To return the immune system to its normal healthy state, the toxins must first be removed. This is what detoxification is all about.

Through the use of all-natural therapies such as diet, supplements, homeopathy, herbs, and glandular extracts, the various toxins are released by the cells and are eliminated through the ears, eyes, skin, and respiratory and excretory systems. As a result, the symptoms that would normally be suppressed by conventional drugs and treatment may make a temporary return.

Additionally, detoxification may cause discharges (skin, digestive, respiratory, or urinary) to occur. When toxins and by-products have built up over a lifetime in your dog's tissues, it may take weeks, months, or even longer for the body to fully clean them out and get rid of them. Here are the primary organs of excretion and discharge signs:

- Respiratory system (eye or nasal discharges, coughing, drooling)
- Skin (itching, rashes, eruptions, or discharges)
- Gastrointestinal system (vomiting, diarrhea)
- Urinary system (increase in volume or frequency of urine, change in color or odor of urine)

Mild symptoms in any of these organ systems may be a normal part of detoxification — as long as the dog feels fine and has good energy and a good appetite. However, please contact your vet if the dog also seems ill or if you have any concerns at all. It's always better to err on the side of safety!

So, don't be alarmed if your dog develops mild symptoms, or her current symptoms get a little worse, during detox. As long as her energy and vitality are good, the program is working. Whatever discharge or drainage you see is the result of the body cleansing itself and thus becoming healthier. For example, in a dog with a skin condition that has been treated with a steroid such as prednisone, the condition may return temporarily. However, eventually it will disappear, as the imbalance that originally caused it is corrected.

However, if a symptom appears *and* the dog also has a poor appetite or becomes lethargic, or if two or more symptoms occur at once, that may not be detox. Please seek veterinary care promptly.

Sometimes additional holistic therapy is needed to rebuild the immune system and body and to direct special attention to certain areas. Your holistic veterinarian will guide you in this process.

As with all other healing therapies, detox must be done gently to avoid dehydration or undue stress. For example, a soft stool is a gentle cleanse, whereas frequent or watery diarrhea may dehydrate the patient. Stay in close touch with your practitioner so he or she can be sure that your dog's electrolytes and fluids stay balanced.

When should you worry?
- Any sign accompanied by fever or lethargy

- Weight loss but the dog doesn't feel better
- Persistent vomiting or diarrhea
- Poor or no appetite

If your dog suddenly stops eating or seems truly ill, call your holistic veterinarian as soon as possible. If you are in doubt about your dog's health, go to an emergency veterinary facility for fluids or any other needed treatment, but first try to connect your holistic vet with the emergency clinic; a cooperative (rather than antagonistic) approach will offer the best results for your dog.

CHAPTER 10
PALEO DOG LIFESTYLE GUIDELINES

Congratulations! By now, you've cleaned out toxins from your home, started your dog on the healthy, nutritious Paleo Diet, and discussed the pros and cons of vaccines and other preventive care with your holistic vet. Now what? Here are guidelines for additional steps toward a true Paleo Dog Lifestyle. We need to round out our program in order to meet all of your dog's needs.

PHYSICAL NEEDS

Exercise

We know that you know . . . exercise is a vital component of any health regimen, for both humans and canines. Sure, it's easier said than done, especially if you're not in the habit. Our dogs need exercise, too — it has the same benefits for them as it does for us, sometimes even more.

If you watch a wolf pack on one of those

great nature shows, you'll see that wolves play, and they play often! Play is not just fun but also instructive for pups as they are growing, learning, and practicing the skills they will need later on. It fulfills both psychological and social roles by strengthening the bonds among pack members and providing a release of energy. It's a great thing to play with our dogs: It's quality time, it's exercise, and it's fun for both of you — what's not to love?

A healthy wolf pack runs about 30 miles per day. Moving is what canines naturally do to hunt and protect their territory. Today, not all dogs need to hold a vast territory, but every dog needs to move — from a 2-pound Yorkie to a 200-pound Mastiff. While breeds vary in their exercise needs and capabilities, each dog is an individual, and no one exercise program fits all sizes, shapes, ages, or breeds of dog.

If your dog is already in great shape — good! You're the exception! Just don't forget to warm up and warm down your dog, just like a human athlete does.

On the other hand, if you're like most people, you and your dog are likely *both* in need of some physical fitness. And just as it's recommended that people check with their doctors before starting an exercise program, you should get your dog a checkup and discuss your exercise plan with your veterinarian.

All dogs are individuals with different needs and abilities. Dogs with short noses (Pugs, Pekingese, Bulldogs, etc.) aren't built to handle strenuous exertion; their breathing just can't keep up. A Greyhound or a Whippet, on the other hand, must run; it's as necessary to them as breathing. Simply opening the door so the dog can run around in the yard is not an exercise program. Canine fitness is a team sport; *you* need to be involved!

When starting an exercise program, do it sensibly. Don't just grab your dog's leash next Saturday and drag her on a 5-mile hike. She needs conditioning, just like you do. Unaccustomed stress on joints and muscles, especially for an overweight dog, can lead to serious injury. A dog's loyalty and love will often keep her going long past the point when she's tired. Pay attention to her body language, and don't push her limits.

Your dog's paw pads also need conditioning. If all they ever come into contact with are floors and grass, asphalt and gravel will be just as uncomfortable on your dog's paws as they would be on your bare feet.

Use special caution in extreme weather. Many dogs have had their paws seriously burned by hot asphalt or bruised by ice. In warm weather, be sure to exercise your dog early in the day or after it cools off in the evening. A heavy-coated dog running in hot weather can easily develop heatstroke, which can be fatal. (The same can happen to any dog left in a car in warm or sunny weather. *Never* leave your dog in the car unattended! You'd be surprised how hot it can get inside a car, even one parked in the shade or on a cloudy day. If the temperature is warmer than 70°F, leave the dog at home while you run errands!) Pay attention to smog alerts in big cities. Your dog shouldn't be breathing that stuff either.

While dogs can wear a collar for their ID and license tags, for outings we much prefer harnesses or head collars. They're more comfortable for the dog and give you better control in an emergency. But most important, the pressure of a collar and leash can harm the important structures in the neck, such as the trachea, esophagus, thyroid, major blood vessels supplying the brain, and the major nerves that accompany them. Many holistic veterinarians have reported the resolution of conditions such as hot spots on the front legs, apparent itchiness of the head, face, ears, or feet, and other conditions attributable to nerve irritation or damage, such as wobbler syndrome or forelimb lameness. A training or show collar, if used properly and only when needed, is fine. Use a collar for fashion or for tags, but a harness or head collar for everything else. Of course, any form of restraint can be misused, so learn the technique appropriate for any device.

If you are a runner, then run with your dog; if you walk or hike, do the same. Instead of going to the gym and sweating under fluorescent lights (something that is the complete opposite of what our own Paleolithic ancestors did), find things to do in the daylight hours. Go to bed earlier, get up earlier, and take that walk before breakfast. Find things that are fun for both you and your dog. Check out agility training — you'll be amazed at the variety of sizes and shapes of dogs who have become agility stars! There are dozens of other canine sports to choose from, from Earthdog to Carting to Flyball, that nearly any size or breed of dog can participate in and enjoy.

The secret to the Paleo lifestyle is to just do it. Move your body, and your dog will follow. Your dog is a social animal and wants to be with you and to please you. We have all seen some pretty amazing dogs on TV from time to time who do all manner of things — even surfing and skateboarding. It's time to separate from the TV and computer screen and go for a Paleo power walk!

Special Exercise Considerations

- *Always* take a bottle of purified water with you for you and your dog.
- If your dog is older or has joint disease, don't overexercise. Swimming is a wonderful activity for many dogs. Moderate exercise, especially when followed by a gentle massage, will be greatly appreciated!
- Some experts recommend limiting exercise for giant breed puppies to 15- to 20-minute walks until their joints are fully mature (12 to 18 months of age) to prevent osteochondrosis, a group of painful joint diseases that also affect humans.[1]
- There is evidence that the risk of hip dysplasia may be increased for puppies who go up and down a lot of stairs when they're young. While puppies do need exercise, you may want to use a baby gate to limit access to stairs.[2]
- Never exercise your dog right before

or after he eats a meal. Let him cool down after exertion. Many breeds are susceptible to a life-threatening condition called gastric dilatation and volvulus, also known as bloat. The risk goes way up for dogs who are exercised on a full stomach.

Grounding

We all used to walk barefoot upon the earth. Animals were in constant contact with the earth until they moved in with us and joined us in our modern way of living. Now most of us are missing that direct contact and the wonders of the planet's magnetic field.

It's almost as if we are living on the moon today, because our buildings, our shoes, our cars, our furniture — everything keeps us separate from feeling the dirt, grass, rocks, and sand beneath our toes and paws! Whether we know it or not, we all have a powerful need for this contact, because we are bioelectrical beings living on an electrical planet.

The relationship between inflammation and disease has finally been recognized — and been brought to the public's attention. Free radicals, which cause and perpetuate inflammation, are everywhere across the media, and every health food store, pharmacy, and grocery store sells a vast array of free radical fighters in the form of antioxidants.

Inflammation was previously considered to be the body's urgent response to injury and infection — and acute, normal inflammation is exactly that. But researchers today are concerned with *chronic* inflammation, and/or oxidative stress, which is now known to be the underlying cause of most common health disorders in both people and their companion animals, including cancer, cardiovascular disease, diabetes, and degenerative conditions like arthritis and cognitive decline (senility). The name of these inflammatory processes usually includes the suffix "-itis" (such as arthr*itis*, gingiv*itis*, dermat*itis*, and so on).

But what, besides providing specific supplements and feeding a healthy diet, can we do about it for our Paleo Dogs? The answer is not that difficult, because we live right on the surface of what may be the biggest anti-inflammatory device ever conceived: Mother Earth herself. It's Earth's surface that provides the magnetic field that we were designed to walk upon.

A strong argument can be made that contact with the soil quenches inflammation by allowing Earth's infinite supply of negatively charged electrons to rise up into the body and to ramp down the chronic inflammation and free radicals that are truly killing us. The theory of Earth as an anti-inflammatory is still just a theory, but how else can we explain the way that grounding, or "Earthing," reduces inflammation and stimulates healing on all levels? We need to get our feet out of our shoes and to get our dogs out on the earth, instead of always being separated from it by floors, cars, and concrete. We need to walk upon the Earth's surface again, lie upon it, lean back against a tree trunk as our ancestors once did and many cultures still do! We must assist this process for our dogs and help them too, to reconnect with the earth.

Science understands that chronic inflammation is also a major factor in aging. Can reconnecting with Earth's magnetic field slow the aging process through its remarkable impact on inflammation?

The natural slowdown that occurs in cells and tissues as we advance in age is responsible for an increased risk of disease and death. Part of this process involves the aging of the immune system, characterized by a chronic low-grade inflammatory status of the whole aging organism. This process is called immunosenescence — and has also been appropriately dubbed "inflamm-aging."

The modern preoccupation with drugs and vaccines has replaced treatments that were used for thousands of years to enhance the immune system, such as Ayurvedic therapies and Chinese medicine, including acupuncture. Instead, today's preventive treatments, such as vaccines and topical flea and tick products, burden a dog's body with a toxic overload that can impact his health for the rest of his life. Ultimately, the body simply ceases to be able to deal with this overload.

The Earthing idea is elegantly simple: Contact with the Earth can counteract free radical damage by providing the body with an abundance of electrons. In chemistry-geek terms, *oxidation* means losing electrons, and *reduction* means gaining electrons. You are probably very familiar with oxidation; that's the technical name for processes like rusting and tarnishing. Oxidation is what free radicals do in the body, and the result is inflammation. And just as rust slowly deteriorates iron, chronic inflammation ultimately damages the tissues and organs of the body.

Electrons are the power behind antioxidants, and so they consequently prevent or reduce inflammation. Such effects produce a relaxation effect on your body and your dog's body, and thus a reduction in physiological stress.

Dogs are particularly sensitive to Earth's magnetic energy. Researchers who were curious about the way dogs tend to circle around and around before choosing the exact right spot to eliminate discovered that dogs tend to align their bodies north to south in line with the planetary magnetic field.[3]

Go for a brief walk, barefoot and bare-pawed, when the weather permits — even if it's just on a tiny plot of grass — for a few minutes every day and touch the ground. Some natural stone surfaces will also help conduct Earth's healing ability, and there are also special sheets, pads, and devices that can aid us in accomplishing some indoor "grounding." (See Resources on page 520.)

Modern living is causing an "electron deficiency" that has been overlooked by both doctors and veterinarians. This is a shame, because it not only adds to our chronic inflammation load but perhaps also increases the ravages of aging itself.

Our dogs, especially those tiny ones who get carried around so their paws almost never touch the ground, will be most happy that we are allowing them to make contact with the earth, which will dynamically boost their body's own self-repair and healing mechanisms.

Sunshine

Paleo Dogs, as well as our Paleo ancestors, lived outdoors in the sunshine. But in the past decade or so, science has done its best to make us afraid of sunlight: "Too much sun will give us skin cancer!" As a result of our indoor lifestyle and slathering on sunscreen anytime we might be forced to go outdoors, we're now largely deficient in vitamin D, which is causing or contributing to problems from asthma and allergies to aging.

Dogs don't manufacture vitamin D in their skin like we do, but sunshine still has important benefits for them. Sunshine kills germs. It's helpful for skin infections, and can even kill antibiotic-resistant bacteria and persistent fungal infections. Sunshine enhances mood, increases energy, synchronizes the circadian clock, and may even protect against disease.

Try to get outside in the sunshine with your dog at least once a day for 20 minutes or so.

Restful Sleep

Before the invention of electric lights, our ancestors slept with their domesticated Paleo Dogs in cool, dark caves, with only dying embers from the fire as their night lights.

Artificial light disrupts the mammalian sleep cycle, despite the creative urges you think are beckoning you to stay up late and work. Whether you sleep with your dog or not, it is time to honor our physiology and sleep in sync with seasonal light exposure.

When we violate these natural rhythms, we alter our biological clock, which controls the hormones and neurotransmitters that regulate our physical functions. When we rely on artificial light to extend our days far past sunset, we fool our bodies into living in a perpetual state of summer. When we are out of sync with our natural rhythms, we suffer the consequences. Our internal circadian rhythm needs dark nights for normal melatonin production and needs daylight to signal a new day. Melatonin modulates the immune system, increases the production of white blood cells, and both prevents and treats several types of cancer.[4]

To get the best out of our Paleo lifestyle, we need to respect these natural rhythms. It is critically important for us and our animal companions to sleep in *total* darkness — no streetlights shining through the window, no LEDs on our electronics, no glowing clocks. Even the smallest light — one no brighter than a candle flame — will disrupt sleep and halt melatonin production. And no, you can't just take a melatonin pill and get the same benefits! Protecting the sleep cycle from light will result in better sleep, improved mental health, less stress, and fewer chronic diseases for you, your family, and your pets.

EMOTIONAL NEEDS

Communication
What is referred to today as nonverbal or interspecies communication is a gift that all life-forms share. It is simply the ability of allowing your heart to speak for you instead of your head.

We all have a bit of the Dr. Doolittle in us. We just need to reawaken the skills that we used before we learned to talk. As infants, we communicated in many nonverbal ways, just as the rest of the animal kingdom does. Through nonverbal communication, you can actually begin to see some things through your dog's eyes and become his voice.

If you conversed with animals as a child, you've probably chalked up your own memories of such experiences to an overly active imagination. Perhaps when you were a child, you heard your mother say that she had "woman's intuition" or "just knew something was wrong." Have you ever thought about a certain friend and then that very person called to say, "I was just thinking about you and wanted to say hello"? These are all examples of nonverbal communication.

You can try this right now: With your dog in another room, empty your mind as best as you can of the background chatter (though it's not necessary to be completely void of thoughts). Slow everything down as much as possible and start by listening to what you are feeling. Let your heart fill up with love for your dog and feel how important he is in your life. Think from your heart instead of your rational mind. Close your eyes, and remember details about your dog: the feeling of his coat, his deep, trusting eyes. Try to visualize him walking toward you as if you were watching him on film. Sometimes, the first time you try this, your dog will be by your side before you know it, so happy that you've communicated with him in his own way.

It's very important to always communicate in positive terms — think of what you want your dog *to* do, rather than what *not* to do. When you say, "Don't jump on the couch," your dog sees the image in your mind's eye of him jumping on the couch. He'll think you want him to jump on the couch if you are projecting that picture. He then jumps on the couch — but your yelling at him for doing so sends mixed signals. Give him the command for the behavior you want, such as "Go to your bed." Take him to his bed and praise him for it, to reinforce the positive behavior.

Nonverbal communication often seems to come most easily with other people's animals. It's sometimes difficult to practice with our own pets because we're too emotionally involved with them, but gradually you'll develop proficiency.

Before you touch any new dog you encounter, first ask his guardian if it's okay. Never just put your hand out or start patting an unknown dog; it's disrespectful to both dog and guardian. After obtaining the guardian's permission, then ask the animal's permission, from your heart. If you're not sure, don't do it.

Petting a dog's aura is more subtle and often more acceptable. Using this indirect method in the space around the dog's body is referred to as touching a dog's "etheric double." You can often feel the animal's energy emanating in the space around him. This is a valuable avenue of communication and diagnosis as well, and through it you can offer much healing as you continue to develop your skills, especially when you use love as your guide.

Nonverbal communication can greatly expand your relationship with animals, but some dogs are reserved, just as certain people are. They simply may not want to converse. Don't be discouraged. Trust yourself and proceed with love, imagination, and confidence.

Stress Management

Modern life is stressful. But where did stress come from, and why do we have it? To answer these nagging questions as they relate to our lives and those of our companion animals today, let's use our time machine and travel back to the Paleolithic age. Back then, humans were constantly facing challenges of a very different kind. All around, every day and night, was the ever-present threat of becoming the next meal for a ferocious meat-eater, like a saber-toothed tiger or a cave bear. Our predecessors needed the ability to instantly turn on the fight-or-flight mechanism, or more accurately, "freeze-fight-flight" since the very first phase, which only lasts a fraction of a second, is to freeze and give our senses a moment to evaluate what the problem is and what to do about it. (Think "deer in the headlights.") This is the adrenaline response that we feel whenever we're startled or frightened: Our heart starts beating faster, we breathe faster, our eyes dilate to take in all the visual information we can get, and our muscles tense up, ready for immediate action. When it kicks in, adrenaline stops all digestive and other maintenance functions, makes us fully awake and alert, and gives us a sudden burst of exceptional energy, strength, and endurance.

This fight-or-flight response has its advantages even today when we have to deal with emergencies. We've all heard stories of people exhibiting strength they had no idea they possessed to perform a life-saving task for someone in desperate need of help.

However, today the fight-or-flight response seems to be triggered by practically all of life's stressful events, even those that aren't life-threatening. Suddenly remembering a forgotten appointment, looking at a stack of bills, or even watching the news can cause this involuntary response. However, the adrenaline reaction was never intended to last longer than it took to deal with the danger. When stress is ongoing, a different set of hormones is triggered — also from the adrenal glands — to cope with chronic stress. The primary hormone in the chronic stress response is a steroid called cortisol.

Cortisol, like adrenaline, has wide-ranging effects on the body. It's useful for longer-term stress, like drought or famine. On the downside, it slows wound healing by disrupting collagen and bone formation, increases water loss through the kidneys (causing the classic drink-a-lot, pee-a-lot syndrome), increases hunger, stresses the liver, and shuts down reproduction.

Physicians and veterinarians see stress-related problems on a regular basis. Since our dogs cannot tell us in words how stress is affecting them, they exhibit various emotional, behavioral, and physical signs. These dogs may display a wide range of abnormal behaviors, such as being disconnected, bored, anxious, or aggressive. This is why the Paleo lifestyle is of such importance, because every improvement you make will lead to restoring balance in both you and your dog and will help you to regain control of your response to stress.

Reduce Stress with Music and
Sound Healing

The everyday noises that we live with on a regular basis — from phones, garbage disposals, vacuum cleaners, leaf blowers, lawn mowers, car horns — bombard us from the moment we awake. But don't forget that they also bombard our dogs, whose hearing is not only more developed but is also designed to hear higher-pitched sounds than we do. Like Paleo Dogs of old, wild canines still locate prey precisely by these sounds, fine-tuning their location by the difference in timing and frequency in how prey's sounds arrive at each ear.

Our dogs' immune systems, like our own, can break down amid all the unnatural sounds and stressful disturbing influences we experience daily in our modern world. Soothing sounds counter some of the discordant noise in our environment and thereby calm our dogs and enhance their sense of well-being.

Many have heard the term *white noise,* which describes an audible spectrum similar to white light, which contains the colors of the visible spectrum. We've probably all enjoyed playing with a prism that separates white light into its component colors. Similarly, white noise is a combination of many different frequencies of sound; the end result is a whispery hum that is very soothing. Ocean, waterfall, and gentle wind sounds are very similar to white noise, which is why they are so relaxing.

White noise is frequently used to mask other sounds. For example, when staying in a hotel, we are often annoyed by sounds coming from the rooms above, below, and next door and from the traffic outside. Fortunately, there's usually a way to turn on the room's fan by itself, if you don't want heat or air-conditioning. In fact, any fan (tabletop, box, ceiling, or bathroom) can serve as an excellent white noise generator to help drown out these annoyances. You can download a white noise app for your smartphone that simulates a fan's hum, or you can purchase a sound generator that includes white noise or other soothing nature sounds.

Listening to music or healing sounds has been used for millennia as a healing therapy. Tibetan bells, crystal singing bowls, Gregorian and Buddhist chants, mantras, as well as "overtoning" (vocal harmonics done with the human voice) — these are but a few of the tools still used today to achieve spiritual realization and healing in all life-forms. They can be used to help in the healing of our dogs, as well.

The right kind of music reduces stress, and you and your dogs can experience many benefits by utilizing the healing frequencies of sound. Animal facilities from shelters to dairy barns use music to keep animals calm, healthy, and productive. Animals respond quite favorably to classical music such as works by Bach and Mozart.[5] Some dogs really enjoy harp music. Researchers believe that the music stimulates brain cell activity. You might want to play a CD on a loop to keep your dog content while you are out, but not too loud — dogs' hearing is more sensitive than ours.

If your dog begins to howl or sing along, evaluate whether he is expressing annoyance or pleasure. No one knows exactly what triggers a dog's howling instinct, but high-pitched sounds, such as ambulance sirens, may trigger his strong Paleo instinct to respond. Or, he may be tuning in to his own social network.

You might wish to explore music played on original instruments where the tuning employs other frequencies besides 440 hertz, the standard A (the note that symphonies tune to before a concert).[6] If you have musical instruments, try tuning them so A is at 432 hertz, and see if you can tell which one your dog prefers. Whatever soothing sounds or music you choose, it should be enjoyed by your whole family!

MENTAL NEEDS

Behavior and Training

The most important aspect of early Paleo Dogs, the one thing that put them on the long road to domestication, was their behavior — more specifically, their behavior with respect to humans. As pack animals, the wolves that first engaged in a relationship with humans already had the social skills and personality traits that would ultimately make them humankind's best friends.

Wolves are wonderful parents. They teach discipline through love, and they earn their pups' respect as well as their packs'. Pups are also very good at emulating adult behavior; thus, they learn their hunting skills as well as their social and communication skills. As each pup matures, he or she finds a place in the pack hierarchy, and this allows harmonious functioning as both hunting and family units.

Today, a dog's behavior (such as aggression or inappropriate elimination) could lead to an early demise as surely as a life-threatening disease or accident. Having a well-behaved dog is an essential part of the human-dog relationship.

If you haven't already, we recommend that you and your dog attend basic obedience classes. Not only will you both learn something new, but these sessions will help create a mutual respect and a deeper bond as well. These classes aren't just for puppies; newly adopted adult dogs as well as dogs who have "slipped" in their responsiveness to your commands will also benefit.

Obedience is more than a series of commands. You must demonstrate clear leadership — that is, create in your dog the desire to do what you ask of him. The result is that your dog will do what you tell him, where and when you tell him to do so, and for as long as you say he should. Learning, pleasing, and being rewarded are some of the things your dog loves best.

We can learn so much about behavior from a really good mother dog. She trains, praises, corrects, feeds, grooms, and relates — 24 hours a day. And it all translates as love to her little ones. Dogs never grow up thinking, "I hate my mother and it's all her fault!"

There is an economy to what a mother dog does. She rarely has to repeat a command or reprimand. She doesn't just talk and cajole, as most humans often do, or ask what her little ones want to do. She makes the decisions, and she enforces her actions. Her patience is vast, but when it gets down to taking care of business, she knows exactly what to ignore and what to correct. She has perfect timing. In just a few weeks, she accomplishes miracles that you, as your Paleo Dog's new parent, shouldn't let your new puppy or dog forget. Do as your dog's mother did: Teach and love at the same time, but don't forget your role as guide and arbiter. Whether you're male or female, you are now "Mom." You must encourage the behavior you want and discourage the behavior you don't want.

The dog's pack instinct survives and harkens back to the Paleo period, whether your dog was bred to point, retrieve, hunt, protect, or just look adorable. Your puppy nuzzled under his mother's chin for attention and affection just as he does with you.

When you attend obedience class or practice what you have learned at home, you'll see the delight your praise, both verbal and physical, brings to your dog. Words are just words, but when there is love and intent behind, hearing your pleased "Good dog!" will make him happy. Don't go too far with praise and get him overexcited — that's not a behavior you want to encourage, cute as it may seem when the dog is young. For good behavior, a warm "Good dog," a loving pet or scratch behind the ear, and loving eye contact, or even a smile that comes from your heart, will go a very long way with your canine friend.

When a puppy does an unwanted behavior, it's perfectly okay to say "No!" or "Out!" (which sounds a lot like mom's reprimanding bark) in a low voice. You don't want him to get the idea that his name is "No!" The idea is to get the dog's attention and redirect him to behavior you prefer.

Just remember, when you need to make a correction, think like his mom did. When Mom corrects, it's always for a behavior she has observed, not for something that happened 2 hours or 2 days ago that was just discovered. Dogs live in the moment right here and now. Reward only good behavior, and reward it immediately to reinforce it.

Operant Conditioning: How All Animals Learn
The basic principle behind "operant conditioning" is the fact that all animals act out of one of two desires: "avoid bad things" and "approach good things." Until the past decade or two, dog trainers emphasized the first part through aversive or negative

reinforcement. Dogs learned what *not* to do by being reprimanded, dominated, or punished when they did it. Fortunately, the misguided "alpha dog" method is on its way out, and "positive training" has become the new standard. In this philosophy, the dog learns because you show her what to do and reward her for it when she does it. Unwanted behaviors are redirected; the human behaviors that inadvertently reward bad behavior are changed; and the dog becomes a happy, willing companion.

While we don't agree with all of Cesar Millan's dog-training techniques, one thing he does very well is point out how the inconsistencies in human behavior create canine "misbehavior." Most of what we don't like about our dogs actually comes from us, even though we don't mean it to happen.

For example, you come home from work and greet your new puppy with great enthusiasm, patting him and talking in a high-pitched voice. He bounces and licks you, and you think it's adorable. But when he grows a little, all that jumping up and mouthing of your hands may get to be unpleasant. You may scold or push him, but remember who taught him that behavior to start with — you're the one who rewarded him for it! Now you need to reward him for sitting quietly and behaving politely.

One good trick for breaking that initial excitement and jumping up is to turn around. Put your back to the dog. He will try to come around in front of you and try again; so you keep turning, and turning — always keeping your face away from him. No eye contact, no voice. Just quietly turn away. Most dogs will give up in less than a minute when they aren't being actively rewarded for the behavior by being given attention (even if it's yelling or pushing — it's all attention to your dog!). Okay, it may take 2 minutes for really stubborn cases! The minute he stops, *that's* the moment to reward him: Praise him with a sincere "Good dog!" and a gentle pat.

In the future, then, when you come home, you should say hello to the dog but not get him all wound up; expect good behavior, and your dog will provide it as long as he understands what you want.

Please understand that physical punishment is inappropriate for your dog. Negative conditioning is part of operant conditioning, but to be effective, it must meet several conditions:

- It must occur immediately (within 2 to 3 seconds of the behavior). Rubbing your dog's nose in a pee accident that occurred hours before does not make your dog understand he should not pee there. It only confuses him, makes him frightened of you, and diminishes your bond with him.
- It must occur every time the behavior occurs, 24/7. If the behavior sometimes happens while you're at work, or in the shower, or asleep, or just not paying attention, punishment just won't work.
- It must be consistent and never be abused.

For almost any unwanted dog behavior, you cannot fulfill these criteria. Remote aversive devices like electric fences may be useful in some cases, but devices like anti-bark collars border on outright cruelty.

The best way to train is with positive reinforcement and by giving your dog acceptable alternatives to the unwanted behavior.

Remember that, in spirit, you are your dog's guardian and caregiver, not his "owner." Your dog is his own being, totally unique. He is not your slave. He is your friend, and you want him to want to be with you because he loves you, not because you own him and he has no choice.

Using a clicker is a great way for you to learn about timing and for your dog to learn a little patience. Clickers are inexpensive and can be found at any pet supply store. The idea is to pair the click with a reward (a small food treat can work very quickly). Once the dog learns that the click means good stuff, you can associate the click with the wanted behavior. This is exactly what happened with Pavlov's dogs — the dogs learned that the sound of a bell always accompanied meals, and eventually the bell alone would cause them to salivate in anticipation. You click as soon as you see the desired behavior (which may simply be the lack of the unwanted behavior!). For a chronic barker, you click and reward whenever he pauses, even for just a second or two. But your timing must be perfect; if he starts barking again before you can click, don't click! Only click when he is quiet. It seems tricky, but once you get the hang of it, it couldn't be simpler or more effective. Clicker training can be used on any animal — although people might look at you funny if you use it on your kid!

Finally, always be gentle and include lots of love in your sessions. This is the magical ingredient in all holistic therapies.

Six Training Tips for Your Paleo Dog

1. Invest in professional training or obedience classes. Begin training when your Paleo Puppy or Paleo Dog has transitioned well to the Paleo Dog Diet, because you want him to be as healthy and happy as possible before you commence training. Do not begin formal training until your puppy is at least 6 months of age and, preferably, is neutered or spayed and well healed from the surgery.

2. Develop your connection and bond by taking your dog with you on foot and in the car as often as possible (of course, never leave your dog in the car in weather that is too hot or too cold). Incorporate training lessons in practical settings that mirror your daily life. What a puppy does at the obedience class may not be what he needs in real life, which is full of distractions. We want our dogs to listen to us, so set him up

for success.

3. Study nonverbal communication. Communicate visually in positive terms. Don't say, "Don't sit on the couch." Rather, say and show your dog exactly where you do want him to sit. Dogs think in pictures, so, through visualization, show the dog the picture in your mind's eye of what you want him to do.

4. Your training should involve your dog's "job" (see "Paleo Dogs Need a Job!" on page 306). If you want him to protect the property, then take him for a walk around the property. Say to him, "Is everything okay here?" Then watch for his re-action. Do the job with the dog so he understands that it is his job to protect the family property.

5. Be consistent. Your dog needs to trust you, and he *will* trust you if you do what you say, and mean it.

6. Don't be afraid to ask for help if you need it. Aggression, especially in puppies, can turn dangerous. Do not try to deal with aggression on your own; seek a qualified profes-sional who has a good track record of success with your dog's particular

issue, whether it be food aggression, leash-related aggression, or any other form. Never meet violence with violence; tapping or shoving an aggressive dog is a good way to earn a visit to the emergency room or worse — plastic surgery comes to mind! Dogs have very sharp teeth that can do a lot of damage. Get help immediately at the first sign of aggression in any dog. If the problem is allowed to go on, it may not be fixable.

Paleo Dogs Need a Job!

Before domestication, wolves had to work in order to survive. Like lions and hyenas, wolves developed a cooperative hunting technique to bring down larger prey, providing more food for more wolves. Their social bonds were also extremely strong.

As dogs and humans evolved together, they made each other's lives better because of their respective jobs. Today, many dogs continue to serve humans by performing various functions, such as hunting and herding, but many more dogs are faced with too many idle hours. How can we serve them now and give them back a job to do? How can we help them feel needed and fulfilled, without them thinking their name is "No!" or "Bad Dog!"

The very first job we can give our dogs is obedience work, which we should teach them for their own safety: to walk on lead, to sit/stay on command, to come, to retrieve. Then we can look to their breed or tendencies to guide us to those behaviors that they have been chosen for over the generations: agility training, dog shows, obedience trials, herding, and sports such as disc dog, musical freestyle, etc. There really is no limit as to what the dog can do if she is stimulated by the teaching you provide. She loves to be with you, loves your praise and your touch. All you need to do is find ways to channel her energies into something productive.

Once your dog understands the basics, you can expand on her leash-walking activities by teaching her to bring you the leash. If she doesn't have issues with shredding paper, fetching the mail or the newspaper could be a responsibility she would enjoy. If she constantly carries a ball in her mouth, maybe she could carry a small bag when you take out the trash or could bring your purse in from the car. Perhaps she could be taught to pick up her toys and put them away. Your imagination is the only limit on what your dog can do! Teaching your dog to carry out her own responsibilities will create an even deeper human-animal bond, which will allow your dog to feel like an important member of her family pack.

CHAPTER 11
PALEO-COMPATIBLE THERAPIES

Throughout this book, we have tried to emphasize the fact that many dogs are not healthy enough today to transition straight into the Paleo Dog Diet and Lifestyle. Some dogs need — and most could benefit from — one or more healing therapies to prepare them for that more natural canine life.

Conventional medicine is often lousy at preventing and treating chronic disease; in fact, it's modern medicine that has created and perpetuates so many diseases. But this is where alternative medicine performs superbly, with its emphasis on healing the whole body from within, rather than on suppressing symptoms. Some holistic modalities are better suited to the Paleo philosophy than others. For example, herbs and hands-on healing would probably have been available to the earliest Paleo Dogs, and our dogs today can certainly benefit from them.

On the other hand, modern living has created so many novel hazards and bizarre complications to the natural Paleo lifestyle that we may need to consider using more advanced or technological methods of healing. Obviously, medical treatments like antibiotics, cardiac pacemakers, and dental surgery weren't available to the first Paleo Dogs; but today, Western medicine definitely has its place. If your dog breaks a leg, it would be inappropriate to waft a sprig of lavender around his nose to calm him without also setting or stabilizing the fracture. In fact, conventional medicine is extremely good at handling emergencies. In an emergency, it's definitely wise to seek appropriate veterinary care.

In this chapter, we will introduce some important concepts about where disease comes from and how to treat it with Paleo-compatible therapies. We have studied and personally used many of them, and we believe that these are the safest and most effective treatments of the hundreds of alternatives out there.

Note: Please consult your holistic veterinarian before embarking on any course of treatment. These therapies should not be used in isolation; supporting the whole body with nutrition is a necessary first step in healing.

THE NATURE AND PROGRESSION
OF DISEASE

Disease begins as a disturbance in the body's energy field. The science of epigenetics makes it clear that experiences, emotions, and beliefs have a profound effect on any organism, including animals and people. While we can't always control what happens in our lives, we absolutely can control how we respond to events that do occur. And, of course, our dogs are very sensitive to the energies we are emitting; our stress becomes their stress, and many times our illnesses become theirs as well.

Our overall health depends on the health of our cells, and our cells operate according to the environmental signals they receive. If a body is flooded with toxins, or even natural compounds like cortisol, cells will be affected. If these signals persist, cells will start to function improperly or even die. The body is now unhealthy, and therefore more susceptible to disease-causing factors, such as bacteria or viruses. When the number of malfunctioning or dead cells is high enough, disease becomes overt.

Signs of illness are simply the visible manifestation of the body's attempt to heal itself, and they appear relatively late in the disease process. For instance, when a virus infects the respiratory system, the body produces lots of mucus to wash away the virus particles. Inflammation flares as the body's defensive white blood cells rush to the area and release chemicals to kill the invaders. A fever may develop in order to kill fragile respiratory viruses that can survive only at normal body temperature. These symptoms may be uncomfortable for the dog, and certainly distressing for you to see, but they are all part of the body's normal defensive and healing processes.

If you give the dog drugs to suppress the symptoms, these normal defenses will be inhibited. The body then has to find another way to combat the infection, which often results in a new symptom. For instance, if a decongestant is used to dry up the mucus and tears, the virus may be able to penetrate deeper into the lungs. Mucous membranes will swell, and white blood cells will congregate, resulting in a deep cough to expel the debris. If we then use another drug to get rid of the new symptom — the cough, for example — the body will continue to search for other ways to deal with the problem. If, say, a cough suppressant is given at this point, inflammation may develop in the lungs that can lead to pneumonia or even asthma.

To return the system to a normal, healthy state, whatever caused the problem in the first place must first be dealt with. In this case, the virus must be killed, and cellular debris resulting from the battle between the immune cells and the virus must be cleaned up and removed. Then the underlying energetic cause — such as diet, vaccine-induced disease, toxic environment, and so on — must be addressed in order to effect a complete cure.

Conventional veterinarians are not trained to produce a real cure for chronic diseases; they are largely limited to suppressive or palliative drugs or surgical means of stopping symptoms. In fact, the goal of conventional medicine is usually to put a stop to symptoms (which appeases the guardians), rather than to effect a real cure at the deeper levels of terrain and energy where disease really starts.

First let's understand that disease follows a pattern; to achieve a real cure, we must proceed back through each step of disease progression to reverse its effects.

Energetic imbalance: Your dog seems fine, and there aren't any symptoms; you may just feel that something's wrong.

In holistic terms, an energetic imbalance is where all disease begins. This disturbance first impacts the mental and emotional level. You may see this as a subtle change in attitude or behavior in your dog. An energetic imbalance always precedes physical symptoms. (See "The Energetic Body" on page 316.)

Functional changes: If the disturbance is treated right away, even severe symptoms may resolve quickly or be avoided. At this point, a conventional veterinarian may not be able to diagnose the problem. For example, your dog is asking to go out more frequently but not straining to urinate, and the urinalysis is normal. Clearly, something has changed, but it's very mild or very early in the disease process, such as the subtle signs of internal imbalance listed in Chapter 1.

Inflammation: If the disturbance remains untreated, inflammation shows that the body is trying its hardest to rebalance itself. At this stage, the dog has a visible problem or clearly feels unwell, often with fever, redness, or swelling; however, if the symptoms are internal, it may not yet be possible to pinpoint where or what the problem is.

Pathology: Finally, the body tries to deal with the problem by moving into pathology, such as bladder stones, thickened skin, or fluid accumulation in the abdomen or chest.

Once this stage has been reached, a cure takes longer to achieve, if it's even still possible. The dog must work his way back through the previous stages of the disease: inflammation, functional changes, and energetic imbalance. This is why it often seems as though the dog is worsening before improving. When a chronically ill dog is given the appropriate treatment, there will often be an immediate mental and emotional response, such as more energy or a better appetite, even though the final "physical" cure may take much longer.

If the pathology is too deeply established, a cure may not be possible. However, holistic therapies can extend life and certainly improve its quality. Terminally ill animals who are treated holistically often feel good for quite a long time, but they tend to "crash" abruptly when the disease finally gains the upper hand. But isn't this better than a long, lingering decline, with your dog feeling a little worse every day? Wouldn't you rather feel great right up until the end, and then release this life quickly, with an absolute minimum of suffering? We would!

Nevertheless, a cure can be achieved by holistic methods in many cases where allopathic medicine offers only a quick (and often temporary) fix. Drugs and other modern methods of treating disease are not Paleo, to say the least, but have nonetheless saved many lives. But the question we want to focus on is this: What can we do instead of suppressive drugs or surgery? Can we use remedies at home that may delay or avert a visit to the vet?

To understand how holistic medicine works, we must delve a little deeper into the energy structure of all living beings, including our dogs.

THE ENERGETIC BODY

Even as hunter-gatherers, humans began to realize that there was something going on that was beyond their understanding, but not beyond recognition. In fact, thousands of years before the agricultural revolution, the development of language had already given rise to what we now call religion. Paleo-era ritual burials are evidence of a belief in the afterlife, which implies something that transcends the body — an animating spirit.

The invention of writing quickly generated written religious works, such as the Hindu Vedas. These ancient texts describe the energy system of the body, and the energy centers, or chakras, that are associated with certain primal sounds ("bija" or "seed" mantras), as well as the colors of the rainbow. Interestingly, treelike energy structures and rainbow colors are common themes in many early religions.

An important concept associated with Hinduism (but expanded to many other traditions) is the aura, an electromagnetic energy field that surrounds, encompasses, and permeates all living things (i.e., a halo). It includes the physical structure as well as its energetic outer layers. Although the aura's structure varies somewhat in different traditions, in general it is made up of four bodies: the physical body (and just above it, the etheric body or etheric double, where some suggest past life experiences may be stored), the emotional body, the mental body (two layers: higher and lower), and the spiritual body (three layers: higher, middle, and lower).

There are seven major energy centers, known as chakras, in the body, beginning with the first (root) chakra at the base of the spine and moving up the body to the seventh (crown) chakra at or a little above the crown of the head. There are also at least five minor chakras, at the hands/feet/ paws, and at the base of the skull (foramen magnum), where the brain stem meets the

A DOG'S AURA

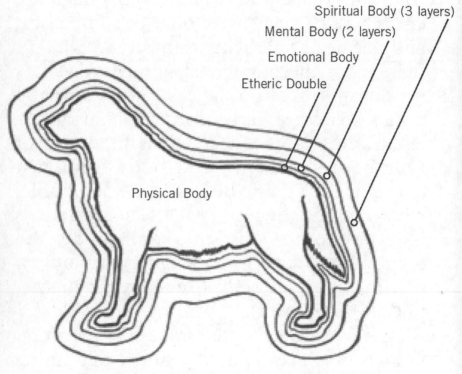

Spiritual Body (3 layers)

Mental Body (2 layers)

Emotional Body

Etheric Double

Physical Body

The etheric double is the nearest nonphysical level.

spine. It is said that as we spiritually evolve, new chakras emerge. The chakras are conceptualized as spinning wheels of light (*chakra* means "wheel" in Sanskrit) in the colors of the visible spectrum.

A specific color is associated with each chakra and can be used to stimulate, sedate, or balance the chakras and their associated organs. Color therapy — the use of light and color in healing — dates from ancient times. You can use colored lightbulbs to bathe your companion in the desired hue, or use colored cloth such as a bandana or bedding. Crystals or stones of the needed color can be placed on or around your pet or added to a collar.

Included in each chakra description below are suggestions for various colors and/or colored stones, gems, and crystals that have been used throughout the ages to promote the healing response.

Chakras and Associated Colors and Gemstones

First chakra (base of spine/tailhead): **Red** stimulates the immune system, increases inflammation, fights tumors, builds the blood, and has an antiviral effect. It relates to the reproductive system and the survival

THE MAJOR CHAKRAS AND THEIR COLORS

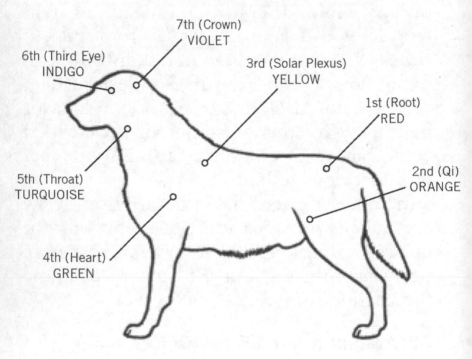

6th (Third Eye)
INDIGO

7th (Crown)
VIOLET

3rd (Solar Plexus)
YELLOW

1st (Root)
RED

5th (Throat)
TURQUOISE

2nd (Qi)
ORANGE

4th (Heart)
GREEN

instinct. As the root, this chakra is sometimes associated with the color black. (Red Jasper, Garnet, Ruby, Hematite, Obsidian)

Second chakra (sacrum, below navel): **Orange** stimulates the appetite and supports the lungs. It also stimulates the thyroid gland and supports milk production. (Carnelian, Orange Calcite)

Third chakra (solar plexus): **Yellow** balances the endocrine (hormone) system and supports the gastrointestinal tract, including the liver and gallbladder, as well as the kidneys and adrenal glands. It is the seat of the fight-or-flight response. (Citrine, Topaz, Tiger's Eye, Yellow Calcite)

Fourth chakra (heart): **Green** soothes and stabilizes energy. It is the most healing color and is especially useful for infections. It is no coincidence that hearts and love are linked together; love is centered in and emanates from this chakra. Pink is also associated with the heart chakra. (Green Aventurine, Jade, Emerald, Malachite, Watermelon Tourmaline, Rose Quartz, Rhodochrosite)

Fifth chakra (throat): **Blue** is anti-inflammatory and is good for wounds and fevers. Blue is a very cooling and sedating color. A combination of green and blue (turquoise) is very restful and helps soothe all kinds of irritations, whether physical, mental, or emotional. (Sodalite, Sapphire, Blue Calcite, Blue Lace Agate)

Sixth chakra (third eye/brow): **Indigo,** a dark purplish-blue color, is associated with intuition, instinct, and insight. It governs the senses and the nervous system. This chakra is highly developed in dogs, and is especially active in guide and therapy dogs. Interspecies communication takes place through this spiritual portal. (Lapis Lazuli, Azurite, Amethyst)

Seventh chakra (crown/above head): **Violet** supports the part of the immune system that produces white blood cells, especially the spleen. Purple is used as a royal color for good reason: It denotes high spiritual advancement in humans. This chakra is also represented by clear or white light. (Amethyst, Purple Fluorite, Diamond, Clear Quartz)

HANDS-ON HEALING

Touch therapy, or hands-on healing of any kind, is soothing and beneficial for our dogs. It helps us communicate and strengthens our bonds with our animal companions.[1] Always approach your dog with honor and respect. Never force an animal to accept any hands-on work — let him tell you how much is okay with him, and for how long.

Here's what many touch therapists recommend: Hold your hands, if your dog will allow it, on any one of the seven chakras or on a painful spot. Relax, and allow positive healing energy to flow from you through your right hand into your dog, and let any negative or painful energy flow from the dog into your left hand and out through your head or feet. (If you are more comfortable using the opposite hands, that's fine, too; just creating the circuit is the important part.) When you're finished, be sure to shake your hands to release any leftover negative energy from your body. Let the dog rest comfortably and use this healing in his own way.

REIKI — UNIVERSAL LIFE FORCE ENERGY

Profound healing is possible through the power of touch. The Reiki practitioner, an initiated individual, channels energy to heal the sick.

Reiki originated in Tibet thousands of years ago, but the technique was lost until 1922, when it was rediscovered by Dr. Mikao Usui of Japan; his students later brought it to the United States.

Reiki is universal energy; it doesn't involve

the energy, clarity, or healing ability of the practitioner. Thus, no negative energy may be absorbed by the healer or transferred from the healer to the subject.

To become a Reiki practitioner, the individual goes through a series of classes and "attunements" that initiate the student and set the Reiki energy pathways, which remain active for life. Universal energy flows in via the crown chakra, through the individual's chakra system, to his or her hands, and thence to the being or object being healed. Whenever an initiated individual touches with intention, the Reiki energy automatically flows through his or her hands, with no effort or expenditure of personal energy. The Reiki initiate is a passive but reliable conduit for healing life energy.

Reiki has three levels:

First-degree Reiki activates the healing energy so that it flows by physical touch or across a short distance; this is useful for animals who do not want to be touched but will accept the energy if the practitioners' hands are a short distance away.

Second-degree Reiki teaches the basic symbols that activate the energy for healing at a distance, without physically being present.

Third-degree or Master-level Reiki attunes

the practitioner so he or she can set the Reiki pathways in another individual, allowing the Reiki master to teach and initiate others.

Reiki may be used on plants, animals, people (from babies to elders), and even on mechanical objects such as cars, washing machines, and computers. It has been shown to be effective in treating everything from mild imbalances to life-threatening illnesses. Reiki is an approved therapeutic practice in nursing[2] and patient care.[3]

APPLIED KINESIOLOGY

Applied kinesiology ("AK" or "muscle testing") is a form of biofeedback that can be done without a machine or technical training.[4] In AK, the body's energy balance is tested by applying stress to certain muscles to gauge the strength or weakness of the spine and organ systems. One such system is called Touch for Health, which was popularized by Dolores Krieger and Dora Kunz in the 1970s.

When the body is stressed, our immune system is impaired, and we are out of balance. To see whether you (the "testee") are in balance using applied kinesiology principles, do the following exercise with a partner ("tester"). First, you and your partner must get into balance, and then you can "surrogate" test your dog.

Simple Muscle-Testing Procedure

- Metal can interfere with testing, so remove all rings, necklaces, watches, earrings, and any other metal from the body. (Inert metal implants like bone pins or artificial knees are okay.) Of course, you shouldn't have your smartphone in your pocket, either!
- Testee (the person being tested) stands in an area that provides 16 inches of clear space all around — away from walls and furniture.
- Testee holds left hand at side and holds right hand out and parallel to the ground.
- Tester (the person doing the testing) faces testee and places two fingers of the left hand on the testee's right wrist.
- Tester tells testee to "hold" (engage the arm muscles) and then presses down gently but firmly (see figure). Don't try to force it; just give a little push.

There will always be a little "give" in the muscle, but if the testee is in balance, the muscles will lock, and the arm will stay "strong" and not be pushed down. If the testee has an energy imbalance, then even if the testee tries hard to hold it up, the arm will go down easily.

To get back into balance, resume the testing position. The tester places two fingers of his or her left hand over the thymus gland (located under the breastbone at the top of the rib cage, which is in front of the heart and behind the sternum) and pushes down on the testee's right wrist; it will usually go down. The testee should then "thump" (a little tap with two fingers) the thymus three times and the tester should then advise the testee to place his or her tongue behind the upper front teeth and keep it there. Repeat. The tester should retest the testee, who should now have a strong right arm; if not, perform the "thymus thump" again. Now, exchange places and repeat until both tester and testee are in balance. Keep in mind that if results are not fruitful that this is not an exact science, and space does not permit for a full discussion on this testing method. Your holistic consultant may be able to demonstrate this procedure in person.

AK testing can be performed for any food, drug, supplement, or even grooming product by having the testee hold the object in

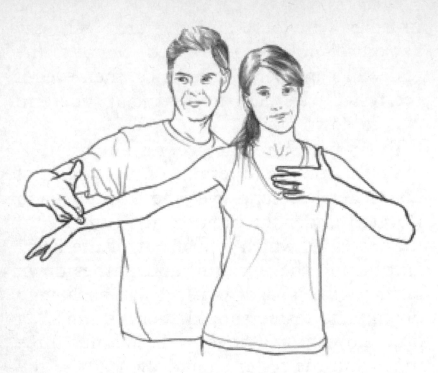

the non-testing hand or by putting each item in a bottle or plastic bag.

Hold the item to be tested in the left hand at the level of the solar plexus (in the triangle formed by the lowest ribs, where your "six-pack" is — or would be if you had one). Many believe that energy enters a body from the left side and exits through the right. Hence, the left arm holds the product, and the right deltoid muscle is tested.

As a fun but powerful demonstration — and to get a feel for the technique — you can put a teaspoon of white sugar or white flour into a bag; these universally test weak for everyone.

- Tester faces testee and places two fingers of the left hand on the testee's right wrist.
- Tester tells testee to hold and presses down on the testee's wrist.
- The arm shouldn't move much if the food/product is beneficial to the subject. Food or products that test strong (meaning the arm doesn't go down) are in balance with the testee. When something tests weak and the arm goes down, the testee's energy is depleted, meaning that the item is not in harmony with the subject at that time. However, the response may change over time. Repeat these tests throughout the day when testing food or supplements. If you test an orange right after you drink a glass of orange juice, for example, you may get a different result than if you test many hours later.

Now, you can test products with your dog. In this case, the testee is also the surrogate. When the surrogate and dog are in physical contact, the tester can read the energy of

329

the dog.

The dog should sit or lie down by the testee's nondominant side. The testee holds the product in the nondominant hand and touches it to the dog's body (anywhere except the head). Testee raises and extends the other arm for testing. If the arm tests weak, the product is not resonating with the dog at this time.

You may also use AK as a diagnostic tool by asking yes-or-no questions. You can even question the remedies or therapies you are considering using. Start each session with one yes and one no question to which you know the answers ("My name is _____" or "I live on Earth"); this will help you make sure your energy is aligned for testing.

If you're by yourself or out in public, there are several "solo" ways to perform AK, such as the "O," or "Ring," technique. Make an "O" with the thumb and finger of one hand, and use one finger of the other hand to try to break the "O." Keep trying — it takes some practice for this technique to become reliable. You can also use a pendulum. Just keep testing often with whatever method that you like and that gives you good results.

Once you have the hang of it, you can test just about anything your dog comes in contact with to determine sensitivities. One little tip: Don't prejudge or have any attachment to the answers. It will put you out of balance, and your results won't be reliable. Just try to be a clear conduit for your dog.

MASSAGE

Giving your dog a massage with loving intent is a wonderful way to improve your bond. Your dog's Paleo ancestors massaged each other consistently with their tongues as a method of grooming, bonding, and providing comfort.

It doesn't take much more than a little stretch of the imagination to empathize with just how good it feels for dogs to be massaged with loving hands, just as it does for us. Be sure your dog has received veterinary care if anything seems out of the norm, and do not apply anything more than light, gentle pressure to the muscles and soft tissues — not the bones themselves, as this will most likely be uncomfortable for your dog and he will let you know it. Err on the side of caution. Consult your vet if your dog is on medication or recovering from a specific injury, and be respectful of his age and condition. Dogs are individuals, and some may love the massage you offer, while others may reject it entirely. *Respect* is the operative word! Never force the issue.

Here are signs that your dog is enjoying a massage:

- A softening in facial expression, especially the eyes
- Sticking the tongue out a little bit and making soft little smacking noises
- Relaxation of the neck muscles demonstrated by a slight lowering of the head
- A deep sigh

We all know what feels good when someone else touches us. Share that lovely touch that you enjoy with your dog, but keep your dog's size, skin, and thickness of coat in mind when deciding what pressure to apply. Too little is better than too much. Don't just rub or mindlessly scratch the same spot continuously, as this may get irritating after a while.

Here are the benefits a healthy dog will get from massage:

- A stretching of tendons and ligaments, which can help with joint flexibility and muscle tone
- An increase in circulation to deep tissues, which in turn helps eliminate toxins from the body

332

- Help recovering from bruises or injuries to soft tissue, muscle soreness and stiffness, and muscle spasms
- A form of passive exercise, which is especially beneficial for arthritic dogs and dogs with hip dysplasia

Massage creates a special time for you to focus completely on your dog, hopefully without distractions (since your dog spends so much of his time focusing on you). This very special one-on-one time can help your dog's attitude greatly and even be an aid for you when training or working on behavior issues.

There are many excellent books to consult and teachers who offer classes on animal massage (see Resources on pages 524–526), but you may wish to explore some of the following simple massage techniques that are often used with good results.

Effleurage: This is a technique that many of us learned in natural childbirth classes that consists of a series of very gentle clockwise circular motions. If your dog rolls over on his back to show you his stomach, this may be exactly the massage technique he might enjoy if done very gently with your whole hand or just the fingertips. The massage can continue up under his armpits and then continue down all four legs, finishing with a deeper massage in the paws.

Ear massage: Ears, like hands and feet, contain acupuncture points that connect to the whole body. Ears can be massaged in little circles with moderate pressure from your fingers, but only if there is no irritation in the ears. Sometimes your dog will settle into an almost trancelike state from the bliss of having his ears lovingly massaged both inside and out with little circles. The very tips of the ears contain points that can relieve pain; most animals will appreciate your firmly holding the tip of the ear between your fingers for a minute or so.

Neck massage: Remove your dog's collars and tags and work the neck muscles from behind (avoiding the throat), kneading gently. Take your first two fingers and trail them down both sides of the spine, and continue this trailing technique gently all over his back. Your dog will tell you what he likes and what he doesn't; always go with the grain of his fur. Some dogs like their tail rubbed and tugged very gently (if they have a tail, of course!).

PHYSICAL THERAPY

A dog's musculoskeletal system is pretty tough, but injuries and age take their toll. A simple but effective tool for reducing discomfort and regaining function is physical therapy.[5] Techniques include passive movements to increase the range of motion, coordination and balance exercises, application of heat (thermotherapy) or cold (cryotherapy), massage, and hydrotherapy (exercises in a therapy pool, such as walking on an underwater treadmill or controlled swimming). Many cities now have one or more facilities specifically for canine rehabilitation that include a therapy pool, where specific hands-on techniques are available.

FAR INFRARED HEAT

Pain from injury and/or aging affects dogs as much as it does humans. Far infrared pet pads or pet beds contain infrared heating elements that emit deep-penetrating, far infrared rays. These rays may promote bloodflow, which can reduce inflammation and provide pain relief for dogs suffering from strains, arthritis, muscle pain, or joint pain. The pads provide extra warmth and help in the recovery process following surgery or other treatments.

Try using a far infrared dog bed or pad for birthing mothers and puppies, because maintaining their 101°F (38°C) body temperature is of critical importance to building their immune systems. Older dogs enjoy the warmth, too. (See Resources on page 534.)

NEGATIVE IONS

Negative ions are produced in abundance in the atmosphere of mountains and rainforests and by waterfalls, rainstorms, whitewater, and ocean waves. That's part of why these environments make us relax and feel good — and why the air feels so fresh and clean after a hard rain. It certainly feels better being there than being in a high-rise office building under fluorescent lights, breathing recirculated HVAC air.

The metal, glass, concrete, asphalt, and plastic environments we have created for ourselves and our pets contain few or no negative ions. Science has shown that increasing negative ions in the environment is helpful for depression, so why not start increasing those ions in our homes and offices?

Himalayan salt lamps are one means of releasing negative ions naturally into our environment, and they can be placed in strategic places around your home or office to impart negative ions. A salt lamp on the floor may become a magnet for pets, who seem to enjoy resting close by. Negative ions are popping up in unusual places as well, such as in the glazing on paintings, which emits negative ions into the ambient air, as well as in pain wraps, pet pads and beds, and even in soap (see Resources on page 536). It is probably safe to say that negative ions can give us all some positive benefits.

CHIROPRACTIC

The basic principle of chiropractic, both for people and animals, is to correct misalignments, or subluxations, of the vertebrae. These put pressure on the peripheral nerves at the root level, where the nerves branch off from the spinal cord and pass between vertebrae. This "pinched" nerve is usually accompanied by pain but may also cause a functional problem.

A chiropractor works to realign the vertebrae by applying gentle force to the spine, tail, knees, shoulders, and other areas of the body. When a dog's vertebrae are out of alignment, the joint capsules stretch and the surrounding muscles may go into a spasm; this can be very painful.

Prior to making an adjustment, the chiropractor needs to observe how the animal stands, moves his head, walks, and turns, as well as how he behaves or reacts, to determine where soreness occurs. Sometimes the practitioner must work on parts of the body that are already painful to the touch. Learning to give your dog a massage at home between visits will not only be enjoyable to your dog but will also help to make him more relaxed during chiropractic treatments.

It's best to find a practitioner who is certified and trained in veterinary chiropractic. A chiropractor without specific veterinary training may inadvertently do great harm. There are two certifying organizations and hundreds of qualified members around the world that can help your dog (see Resources on page 511).

HERBAL THERAPY

We can't cover herbs in depth in this book; however, we can offer some highlights from this fascinating field. Herbal medicine is very powerful, so we strongly recommend always working with a veterinarian who is comfortable with herbal therapy.

Influenced by ancient cultures, healing systems all over the world today embrace herbalism. The Indians embrace Ayurvedic medicine, which links the microcosm to the cosmos; they commonly include herbal remedies in their medical practices. Tibetans, whose medicine was under the

338

control of the lamas and therefore closely linked to their religion, carefully coordinated the harvest of herbs to coincide with helpful astrological influences. Swiss alchemist Paracelsus subscribed to the doctrine of signatures, which used a plant's outward appearance as an indicator of what it could cure (for instance, nutmeg and walnuts resemble the brain, so they were thought to improve mental abilities).

The Chinese view disease as a sign of disharmony within the whole person. Herbs have been crucial to Chinese medical practitioners since about 2500 BC. Many of their formulas go back thousands of years and were handed down through the generations in herbal dynasties. The five elements in Chinese herbal medicine — wood, water, metal, earth, and fire — form a network of relationships. Each element represents a season, a taste, an emotion, a personality type, and certain parts of the body (for example, fire represents summer, bitter taste, joy, extrovert, and the heart, small intestine, tongue, and blood vessels). The forces of yang and yin and qi (or chi) complement the basic model of the five elements. Yang and yin represent balance; and qi, vital energy.

Herbalists use the bark, berries, bulbs,

flowers, fruit, gum, hips, hulls, leaves, roots, root bark, seeds, tops, and the whole plant — all according to tradition or recipe. Many modern pharmaceuticals are synthetic versions of the active ingredients of herbs. The salicylic acid in aspirin was isolated from white willow bark, cortisone isolated from yucca, and digitalis (digoxin) isolated from foxglove.

Herbs are often sold individually, but most work better in combination. There is a synergy that is created when they are combined. Most herbs shouldn't be given over long periods of time — 3 to 4 weeks at most — because the body seems to build up a tolerance, and they lose their effectiveness. Many herbs do have nutritional value, however, and are taken as supplements.

First, let's take a look at the various ways to administer herbs.

Decoction: A tea made from roots and bark. Gently boil and then simmer 1 tablespoon of cut herb or 1 teaspoon of powdered herb in 8 ounces of water for 15 to 20 minutes, then let it stand for 5 to 10 minutes.

Infusion: A tea made from leaves or blossoms. Boil 8 ounces of water and remove from the heat. Add 1 teaspoon of powdered herb, cover, and steep for 10 minutes.

Extract/tincture: A process that extracts the active and volatile ingredients from herbs into a solvent, such as ethanol, apple cider vinegar, or glycerin. Extracts are liquids, making them easy to assimilate. These formulations are excellent for dogs, and they may be further diluted in water when necessary.

Herbal oil: An extraction of herbs in an oil base.

Fomentation: A cloth soaked in a hot infusion or decoction, wrung out, and applied to an affected area.

Poultice: A moist, hot herb pack applied topically (which is more effective than a fomentation). When using fresh herbs, crush and bruise them. If they're powdered, mix them with mineral water to form a thick paste. Spread them on clean cloth and cover the affected area. Never reuse a poultice; always make a fresh one because they lose their potency.

Caveat: "Natural" does not mean safe. Herbal medicine is very powerful; we strongly recommend working with a veterinarian who is experienced with herbal therapy. That said, there are a few safe herbs you may wish to keep on hand at home in case you need their special properties.

- **Aloe vera:** The inside of fresh-cut leaves can be used to soothe and heal scrapes and burns.
- **Chamomile:** Use in capsules, treats, or as a strong tea to calm anxious or hyperactive dogs.
- **Eucalyptus:** Use fresh or dried eucalyptus leaves in hot water to fill a room with its scent; the steam will help clear sinuses and improve breathing. Never give eucalyptus internally.
- **Ginger:** Give 1/4 teaspoon or 1 to 2 capsules (reduce the dose for dogs under 20 pounds) to prevent motion sickness or to ease nausea.
- **Marshmallow:** Give 30 minutes before meals in capsule form or as an infusion for sensitive stomachs or inflammatory intestinal conditions.
- **Nettles:** Give capsules for skin rashes or allergic skin disease to help reduce histamine release.
- **Turmeric:** Its strong anti-inflammatory properties may be helpful to soothe flare-ups of inflammatory conditions such as arthritis.
- **Yarrow:** Use fresh, mashed leaves as a poultice to help stop bleeding and heal wounds.

Herbal Combination Formulas

We provide the following combination herbal formulas as a convenient reference. These are the formulas most commonly used for common canine conditions. These combinations have been suggested by several herbal experts, but they are not intended as medical advice. Please consult your holistic practitioner prior to experimenting with any medicinal herbs. Even if your veterinarian has recommended one or more herbs, it's up to you to observe your dog for possible adverse reactions. As always, proceed with caution.

You may find combinations for humans at your health food store; most are likely safe for dogs, but they may not be ideal. As a rule of thumb, the oral dosage of herbs on the human market is based on a 150-pound human, so you can use a proportional dose based on your dog's weight. But it's not necessarily a straight conversion: Small dogs may need more of certain herbs because of their faster metabolism, and large dogs may need less. Herbs are powerful medicine, and they may adversely interact with any pharmaceuticals your dog may be taking. We strongly recommend consulting your holistic veterinarian before giving any herbs to your dog, just to be safe.

For respiratory problems and sinusitis, many herbalists combine:

Goldenseal	Natural antibiotic-like herb for congested membranes. Reduces swelling, helps clean system.
Capsicum	Relieves congestion, disinfects, acts synergistically to increase the power of other herbs. (*Note: This is cayenne pepper, which can be extremely irritating; use caution!*)
Parsley	Increases resistance to infection.
Marshmallow	Helps remove mucus from lungs.
Burdock	Purifies blood.
Mullein	Cleanses lungs.

For heart and circulation problems or fatigue, combine:

Hawthorn	Strengthens heart.

| Capsicum | Facilitates the action of other herbs on the heart. |
| Garlic | Natural antibiotic and immune stimulant. |

Additionally, marine-source omega-3 oils, coenzyme Q10, taurine, and carnitine are beneficial for heart problems in dogs.

For digestive upsets, irritable colon, or diarrhea, combine:

Marshmallow	Contains mucilage, which aids the bowel.
Slippery elm	Soothes, draws out impurities, heals, acts as a buffer against irritation.
Ginger	Relieves gas, settles stomach. Give 30 minutes before traveling for carsickness.

In case of diarrhea without other symptoms, such as lethargy or depression, fast the dog for 24 hours to let his system rest and repair. Provide fresh purified water at all times; consider fluid therapy if dog becomes dehydrated.

For blood purifying, cleansing, eczema, ringworm, or cancer, combine:

Pau d'arco	Natural antibiotic, antifungal.
Licorice	Natural expectorant. Supplies energy.
Sarsaparilla	Cleanses, stimulates body defenses.
Cascara sagrada	Effective laxative.
Oregon grape root	Natural antibiotic and tonic for all glands.
Prickly ash	Improves circulation.

For worms and other parasites:

Note: Many herbs and combinations are recommended; however, don't rely on herbs alone. Have your dog's stool checked after therapy to make sure the problem has been taken care of.

Pumpkin seeds	Expel tapeworms.
Garlic	Makes the digestive tract inhospitable to parasites.

Black walnut	Often recommended, but it can be extremely toxic. Do not use without veterinary advice and supervision.

For liver problems, one or more of the following herbs may be helpful:

Red beet	Nutritious for liver.
Dandelion	Stimulates liver.
Parsley	Cleans out toxic waste.
Liverwort	Helps heal damaged liver.
Blessed thistle	General tonic to system.
Angelica	Helps eliminate toxins in liver and spleen.
Chamomile	Helps cleanse toxins from liver.
Gentian	Stimulates liver.
Goldenrod	Stimulates circulation.
Barberry	Causes bile to flow more freely.
Ginger	Acts as a stimulant.
Cramp bark	Good for congestion and hardening of liver.

Fennel	Helps move waste material out of body.
Peppermint	Cleans and strengthens entire body.
Catnip	Strengthens liver and gallbladder.

For kidney, bladder, or urinary tract problems, combine:

Goldenseal	Helps kidneys eliminate toxins.
Juniper	Antiseptic to kidneys.
Uva-ursi	Strengthens urinary tract.
Parsley	Nutritional to kidneys, mild diuretic.
Ginger	Cleanses kidneys.
Marshmallow	Soothing to urinary tract.
Horsetail	Tonifier, helpful for urinary crystals or stones.

Helpful hints: For dogs with calcium oxalate crystals and stones, avoid oxalate-containing foods such as beets (roots and greens), okra, spinach, sweet potatoes, soy, nuts, elderberry, figs, rhubarb, lentils, sesame seeds, and almonds.

For strengthening, stimulating, and cleansing the glands, combine:

Kelp	Contains iodine needed by thyroid glands. (Please check with your veterinarian regarding increasing any iodine, as certain thyroid conditions could be aggravated by an excess.
Dandelion	Stimulates glands, increases activity of liver.

For weight problems, combine:

Irish moss	Purifies and strengthens cellular structure.
Parsley	Overall cleanser.
Watercress	Acts as tonic.

For nervous disorders, combine:

Dill	Soothing to the stomach.
Valerian	Relaxes nerves.
Hops	Contains B vitamins for nerves.
Passionflower	Combines well with valerian.
Chamomile	Calms and soothes.

For bone healing, combine:

Comfrey	Heals wounds, bones. (Use with caution.)
Goldenseal	Natural antibiotic with healing powers. Contains vitamins and minerals.
Slippery elm	Draws out impurities.
Aloe vera	Natural detoxifier. Removes toxic matter from body, heals and protects.

For arthritis or inflammation of the joints, combine:

Bromelain	Reduces swelling and inflammation.

Yucca	Contains soothing saponins.
Alfalfa	Contains alkaloid for pain, and nutrients for body strength.
Black cohosh	Relieves pain, irritation, acid condition of blood.
Yarrow	Cleans blood, helps regulate liver.
Capsicum*	Catalyst for other herbs.
Devil's claw	Benefits rheumatism as well as arthritis.
Burdock	Reduces swelling.

For skin and coat problems, combine:

Alfalfa	Contains trace minerals, which benefit skin and coat.
Burdock	Good for burns and wounds.
Goldenseal	Helps stop itching.

For ear problems:

Diluted garlic oil from a capsule or mullein oil (1 or 2 drops) may be squeezed directly

* This is cayenne pepper, which can be extremely irritating; use caution!

into the ears. Goldenseal and echinacea have natural antibiotic properties that may be beneficial.

For eye problems, combine and take by mouth (do not put in eyes):

Goldenseal	Natural antibiotic.
Bayberry	High in vitamin C.
Eyebright	Strengthens immunity to eye complaints.

For birthing, pregnancy, and estrus (heat cycles), combine:

Red raspberry	Strengthens uterus, regulates uterus during delivery, prevents hemorrhaging, reduces false labor pains.
Blessed thistle	Helps promote flow of milk, eliminates mucus congestion.
False unicorn	Strengthens ovaries, overall tonic for system, rich in trace minerals.
Black cohosh	Helps in uterine disorders.

| Hops | Reduces problems associated with heat cycles, can reduce male sexual tension. |

For fasting, combine clear day chicken broth recipe (see page 246) with a pinch each of one or more of the following herbs:

Licorice	Good for strength and quick energy. Nourishes glands, inhibits growth of harmful viruses.
Hawthorn	Burns up excess fat, strengthens heart, helps insomnia, calms nervous system.
Fennel	Internal anesthetic. Relieves gas, cramps, and mucus accumulation.
Beet	Stimulates and cleans liver, strengthens system.

AROMATHERAPY

Aromatherapy is the therapeutic use of essential oils to heal, nurture, and care for the body, mind, and spirit.

Scent is a powerful component of holistic health care. The subtle use of aromatherapy can enhance all healing therapies, especially for dogs, whose sense of smell is far more complex and acute than our own.

Properly used, aromatherapy stimulates the immune system and promotes healing. These aromatic preparations have many desirable properties that help ease daily stress and aches and pains and assist in recovery from injuries.

The use of scent can be broken down into three different forms:

1. Fresh plants, which contain large amounts of energy in their flowers, twigs, and leaves. Grow your own pet-safe plants, or buy them at health food stores, farmers' markets, and/or organic nurseries. If you plant your own garden, please observe organic principles; sniffing or consuming chemical fertilizers, herbicides, and pesticides can be harmful to a dog.

2. Dried herbs in which the fragile aromatic oils haven't evaporated. Check local herb shops or peruse the shelves of your health food store

for both herbs and spices.

3. Essential oils are volatile aromatic substances that naturally occur within specific plants, such as rose and garlic, giving them their pungent odor. Distilled or expressed essential oils can be purchased at most health food stores.

When our dogs' wild cousins are sick, they seek out certain herbs and plants to munch on or roll in, in order to self-medicate. Some of today's dogs still seek out various plants and grasses for this purpose. However, these are fresh, live plants; aromatherapy oils are highly concentrated in a way the early Paleo Dogs would never have encountered. You may find your new Paleo Dog's tastes becoming more discriminating as you implement each step of the Paleo Dog Program.

Certain essential oils can help our animals because they contain properties that sedate, soothe, or inhibit fatigue, anemia, injuries, anorexia, or infections; they may also be used to control fleas and other pests.

There are several important cautions regarding essential oils:

1. Fragrance oils and essential oils are not the same thing. We are discuss-

ing only essential oils.

2. Use only the best-quality essential oils (see Resources on page 532). Poor-quality or cheap oils may contain all manner of toxic solvents.

3. Avoid any oils high in phenols, such as oregano, thyme, cinnamon (cassia), savory, cedar, birch, and tea tree oil; in ketones, such as sage; in pinenes, such as pine, spruce, fir, bergamot, and eucalyptus; and in limonene, including lemon, orange, tangerine, mandarin, grapefruit, and lime.

4. Also avoid stimulating oils such as ginger, clove, cardamom, rosemary, basil, and mint, unless they are in a highly diluted form like a hydrosol (a water-soluble by-product of essential oil distillation).

5. Never use essential oils straight, or neat; always dilute them into a neutral oil such as almond or olive oil.

6. Essential oils can be very dangerous if used improperly. They should never be applied directly on the skin or taken internally, because they can cause severe allergic reactions, seizures, burns, and even death.

7. Do not force aromatherapy on your dog or confine her in a room where essential oils are being used. Oils that we find pleasant may be quite aversive to your dog. Always give pets an escape route.

Be judicious with your use of essential oils and always dilute them first with a carrier oil (using 5 percent or less of essential oil and the rest carrier oil), such as olive, almond, or sesame oil. Put a few drops of the mixture on your hand, work it in well, and then let your dog sniff it so that you can gauge your dog's reaction. Watch for signs of acceptance, such as sniffing, tail wagging, and showing great interest. However, do not let the dog lick the oil; essential oils are not intended for internal use (unless specifically instructed by your holistic veterinarian).

If your dog dislikes the oil you are testing, the behavior displayed might include turning away, panting, drooling, pacing, whining, sneezing, or snorting. That's a "No!" in no uncertain terms; please honor your dog's decision and do not use that oil.

Do not apply essential oils, even if diluted, to your dog's head, face, feet, or other areas. This is disrespectful, because the dog can't get away from the smell. What smells lovely to us may be overwhelming or even aversive to your dog. As noted, we want to always offer our dogs an escape route from the scent if they so choose.

Essential oils can have a very beneficial effect on shelter, rescue, and adopted dogs by helping the dog bond with the new caregiver after a traumatic experience. The use of a diffuser may be of value, so long as the room where the essential oils are being diffused is well ventilated and offers the dog an escape route. The following oils and combinations may assist in a variety of circumstances:

To lift or lighten mood	Rose
For comfort	Lavender
For courage	Yarrow
To relieve depression	Jasmine, lavender, marjoram
For happiness	Apple, neroli
For healing	Coriander, cypress, myrrh, niaouli, palmarosa, sandalwood, spearmint (hydrosol only)
For infections	Garlic, lavender

For love	Carnation, jasmine, rose (and many others)
To improve memory and impart wisdom	Sage
For peace	Chamomile, rose
For physical energy	Nutmeg, mint (hydrosol only)
For sleep and calming	Chamomile, jasmine, lavender
For calm attention during training sessions	Lavender

Never use artificial or synthetic scents. Like processed food and chemically isolated vitamins and minerals, synthetic oils are missing "life energy" and are useless as aromatherapy. The "good stuff" comes from living things, and thus has a direct link with the earth — a subtle energy that can't be duplicated in a laboratory. The energies of real plant materials merge with our own and those of our dogs to support healing. For example, genuine rose oil envelops us in scent and guides us through a field of flowers, just like the aroma of fresh roses. A synthetic rose oil contains nothing living; it will probably give you a headache and repel your dog.

Good-quality essential oils are always sold

in dark glass bottles (e.g., amber or cobalt) and stored away from light, heat, air, and moisture.

Essential oils should never be given internally. Watch for allergic reactions, and be sure dogs, cats, and children don't have direct access to the oils.

On a similar note, take care with your choice of houseplants, as some are poisonous to pets, who may nibble on them if the scent is attractive. Poisoning symptoms include drooling or foaming at the mouth, vomiting, diarrhea, seizures, ataxia, coma, intense thirst, rapid pulse, swollen mouth and throat, and itching, redness, and blistering of the skin.

TREATING CANCER HERBALLY

Cancer is the most frightening diagnosis of all. Treating cancer requires a carefully planned program, designed in cooperation with your holistic veterinarian. A complete anticancer program will include nutrition, energy therapies, and physical support.

Many herbs are documented to have anticancer properties. Some of the most well-known and widely recommended herbs include the following:

Essiac: This legendary Native American tea is made from burdock root (*Arctium* *lappa*), Turkey (or Indian) rhubarb (*Rheum palmatum* L.), sheep sorrel (*Rumex acetosella*), and slippery elm bark (*Ulmus fulva*). Essiac, also called Ojibwa tea, is often used as a general tonic. It is considered safe, but buy it from a reputable source and follow the directions exactly.

Hoxsey formula: This herbal blend contains red clover (*Trifolium pratense*), chaparral (*Larrea tridentata*), licorice root (*Glycyrrhiza glabra*), Oregon grape (*Mahonia aquifolium*), burdock (*Arctium lappa*), sarsaparilla (*Smilax officinalis*), echinacea (*Echinacea purpurea*), and prickly ash bark (*Zanthoxylum clava-herculis*), plus or minus other ingredients depending on the source. Red clover and chaparral can have serious side effects; do not use except under veterinary supervision.

Carnivora (Venus flytrap; *Dionaea muscipula*): This species of carnivorous plants contains amino acids, quercetin, and other immune modulators that may have cancer-fighting properties.

Graviola *(Annona muricata)*: Studies in humans have shown promise, especially against multidrug-resistant cancer cell lines.

Mistletoe (*Viscum album* L. Iscador): The mistletoe plant itself is highly toxic; however, there are preparations or extracts that are thought to stimulate the immune system, kill cancer cells, and reduce tumor size. Mistletoe is typically used in conjunction with surgery, chemotherapy, and/or radiation because it may help minimize side effects of these radical treatments. Mistletoe herbal extracts are available, but because of their potential toxicity, never use them without close veterinary supervision (see Resources).

HOMEOPATHY

Homeopathy was developed by German physician Samuel Hahnemann in the late 18th century. At that time, people were being treated with poisonous substances to get the "bad humors" out of them by purging (inducing vomiting and/or diarrhea), sweating, and bloodletting. Many patients (including George Washington) died from these treatments.

Dr. Hahnemann developed two fundamental principles upon which he based homeopathy.

1. Law of Similars: If a healthy individual develops certain symptoms when exposed to a substance, similar symptoms in a sick person may

be cured by the same substance.

2. Minimum Dose: Homeopathic remedies are prepared by multiple dilutions of the original substance, along with shaking the dilution in a specific motion called succussion. "High-potency" remedies are the most diluted and succussed, and therefore have the most energy. Practitioners using Dr. Hahnemann's homeopathic system are called classical homeopaths (see Resources on page 534).

In homeopathy, symptoms are important tools, both for determining what remedy is needed and for monitoring the healing process. Homeopaths do not use drugs or remedies to suppress symptoms. This is the opposite of most conventional medical treatments, which are mainly directed at getting rid of symptoms. Homeopaths believe that suppressing symptoms not only thwarts the body's effort to heal but also drives the disease to a deeper — and more dangerous — level. Symptoms are manifestations of the body's attempt to heal itself, so we need to honor them, not rush to eradicate them; they are our windows into the internal process. Homeopathic remedies act in the same way as the natural defense reactions of the body — by stimulating the immune system so it can complete the job it was already trying to do.

Homeopathy uses remedies based on the Law of Similars. When used appropriately, homeopathy works with the body, not against it. The goal is a real cure, not just the suppression of symptoms. In contrast, modern pharmaceuticals work against the body: *anti*-biotics, *anti*-inflammatories, *anti*-depressants, *anti*-seizure, *anti*-cancer. And surgery isn't much better: We remove it completely (appendix, gall bladder, tonsils), whack off parts of it (amputation), or replace it (artificial hips and hearts).

The principles of homeopathy state that there are three possible outcomes of treatment: suppression, palliation, and cure.

- Suppression gets rid of specific symptoms but drives the disease into other channels by denying the body's expression of the original disease. Chemotherapy is an example of a suppressive treatment. As a result of suppression, even though the most troubling symptom is gone, the patient often feels worse overall.
- Palliation means to alleviate symp-

toms; this is how aspirin treats pain. However, for palliation, the medicine needs to be repeated frequently. By treating only symptoms and not the whole individual, allopathic medicine tends to be limited to the first two outcomes.

- Cure, the only goal of homeopathy, means that the body eliminates the whole disease, not just the symptoms, and rises to a state of optimum health. Health is defined as not just the absence of symptoms but also a feeling of well-being and vitality.

Homeopathy is a wonderful method for treating canine imbalances because our companion animals are subtle creatures who live in the moment. When they don't feel well, they don't wish to be fussed with. Homeopathic remedies are easy to administer, are safer than drugs, and give the body a gentle yet powerful nudge to heal itself.

Most conventional veterinarians know nothing about homeopathy and have relegated it to the "quack" category without the slightest understanding of its principles. But homeopathy can truly cure disease, whereas allopathic medicine cannot — and most of the time, doesn't even try.

If your dog has undergone long-term drug therapy, homeopathy may not work immediately. But with patience and persistence, homeopathy may be able to help restore a dog's health, or at least return the dog to a good quality of life, when conventional veterinarians might recommend euthanasia. It's at such traumatic times that homeopathic veterinarians are asked to perform miracles, and many have done so. Very ill animals who are treated homeopathically may not be cured or even palliated, but it may make them feel better. However, you don't have to wait until hope is all but lost — take your dog to a homeopathic veterinarian (or arrange a telephone consultation) as soon as possible.

The exact mechanism by which homeopathy works has not been proven, although we may be getting close.[6] Dr. Hahnemann did "provings" by giving each remedy to healthy people and meticulously recording every effect. Animal lovers will appreciate that Dr. Hahnemann did all of his testing and research on human subjects. Fortunately, homeopathic veterinarians have found that the symptoms in people correspond to symptoms in animals, so our dogs may now reap the benefits of this work.

Working with Homeopathy

A cure in homeopathy involves more than just making the symptoms go away. Rather, it helps the body resolve the underlying cause of the symptoms. Symptoms go away and stay away permanently; the dog feels — and is — healthy in every respect (with none of the symptoms of underlying imbalance listed in Chapter 1). He may still get minor ailments, but he will recover from them with very little or no treatment. When a dog is given an appropriate remedy, you'll often see an immediate mental and emotional response of contentment, even though the final "physical" cure may take much longer. A rough rule of thumb is that it takes 1 month to heal for every year of illness.

It's important to understand that homeopathy is not herbal medicine. Rather, it utilizes medicines derived from plant, mineral, and animal sources. However, we should not think that synthetic medicine is dangerous and that natural medicine is safe. Since homeopathy is powerful enough to cure, it's also powerful enough to harm.

It's difficult for "newbies" to fully grasp the idea that selecting a remedy in haste could cause an aggravation (make the condition worse), palliate the symptoms (cause the symptoms to go away temporarily but later return unchanged), or suppress them (cause the symptoms to go away but make the animal feel worse overall or develop a more serious disease condition later). Allopathic medicine usually palliates or suppresses symptoms, but any modality can do that. It's always best to work with an experienced homeopathic practitioner. Selecting the right remedy in the right potency and knowing when to re-prescribe for a deep, chronic disease is extremely complex.

In homeopathy, remedies are prescribed on the "whole" symptom picture. It would be incorrect to take a remedy to treat a specific ailment.

Homeopathic Remedies to Keep on Hand

While we do not advise trying to treat your dog's deep or chronic disease all by yourself, many minor problems that crop up can be treated at home, such as injuries or acute flare-ups that need symptomatic management until your veterinarian can be contacted. Generally, you will use low potencies (up to 30C), and give one dose every 6 to 8 hours for up to three treatments (unless specifically stated otherwise). If you are not seeing results after the third dose, that remedy is probably not going to work and you should seek veterinary care, whether holistic or conventional.

The following is a list of our top 10 favorite remedies for treating various issues.

Aconite (Aconitum napellus): This remedy is one of the most important in the homeopathic arsenal. Aconite, made from the lovely but highly poisonous plant monkshood, is the first remedy for sudden fear or terror. A dose of Aconite should be given to any animal who has nearly "met his Maker" — narrowly escaped from the wheels of a car or any other situation where a dog would be frightened to death. This intense, deep fear, when left untreated, can result in seemingly minor injuries taking a drastic turn for the worse.

The other major use for Aconite is for any "-itis," or sudden inflammatory, condition. It is great for aborting upper respiratory infections (rhinitis or sinusitis) if given at the first sign of fever or sneezing and may have a similar effect if given early for flare-ups of chronic inflammatory conditions.

Occasionally, Aconite will cure chronic conditions that originally began after a frightening experience. Very high potencies are usually necessary.

Apis mellifica: This remedy, made from the honeybee, is used for problems that are similar to a bee sting, with a lot of burning, redness, and swelling. Usually we think of this remedy for swelling that is unusually intense and is relieved by application of cold compresses. It can be used for insect bites or stings of any kind that have a red and swollen appearance.

It is a good remedy for any condition that is very red and puffy. Apis patients may also be particularly irritable.

Arnica montana: No home should be without homeopathic Arnica, a remedy made from a floral member of the Aster family. It is the primary trauma remedy — essential for bruises, blows, falls, and concussions. It is a good remedy to give after surgery (especially after tooth extractions) to help heal the tissues. In humans we think of it as a sort of "Monday morning" remedy, to ease achy muscles that were overexerted on the weekend. Arnica helps pain that has a sore, bruised feeling.

Arnica is also excellent for healing chronic conditions resulting from old injuries, such as posttraumatic arthritis.

Arsenicum album: This wonderful remedy, made from the toxic metal arsenic, has great application in many conditions. It is the primary remedy for poisoning of any kind, but especially for food poisoning or for those who have eaten something a little "off." Vomiting and diarrhea together often call for Arsenicum. A watery stool, especially with blood, is another indication for this remedy, as are acrid (burning) discharges from the eyes or nose. Pets in an Arsenicum state are usually very chilly, restless, anxious or fearful, and thirsty for frequent, small drinks of water. It is also a major "vaccinosis" remedy — one that can relieve symptoms that are commonly attributed to vaccination, such as asthma or irritable bowel syndrome.

For very ill animals who are nearing death, Arsenicum often provides at least temporary relief of discomfort and may ease their transition as well. Arsenicum in very high potency is sometimes used for euthanasia.

Carbo vegetabilis: This is not a frequently needed remedy, but it does have two very specific applications. One is for breathing difficulty, where the dog seems unable to get enough air (because of asthma, heart or lung disease, or any other condition). The other use is for shock. Severely injured animals will rapidly become shocky — their bodies, especially the extremities, feel cold, and their mucous membranes may be pale and bluish rather than pink. Pets needing this remedy obviously also need emergency medical care, but while you are on the way to the vet, give this remedy every 10 to 15 minutes to help forestall cardiorespiratory shutdown.

Carbo veg is also helpful in cases of known carbon monoxide poisoning.

Ledum palustre: This is the number one bite-wound and puncture remedy, whose origin is the primitive plant club moss. If you know your pet has been in a fight, especially if you find any evidence of a bite wound (but even if you don't), give a dose of Ledum as soon as possible. Ledum will often prevent abscesses from forming if given quickly after a puncture wound. Ledum wounds tend to feel better with application of cold rather than heat. Any insect bite, snake bite, injection, or other deep puncture may also call for Ledum, and it is absolutely essential to give it immediately after having your dog microchipped.

Nux vomica: As you might expect from the name, this is a good remedy for vomiting problems. Known as an excellent hangover remedy for humans, it has great application in dogs for chronic vomiting and suspected ingestion of foreign bodies. (Nux vomica has helped patients expel such delicacies as baby socks and chicken bones, though we haven't tried it for remote controls!)

Nux vomica — which comes from the same plant as the well-known poison strychnine — can be used for spasms or cramping, as well as for constipation. It soothes irritated tummies as well as simply irritable dogs. (Nux patients tend to be very grumpy and want to be left alone.)

Rhus toxicodendron: Here's an interesting remedy from a plant most of us would rather avoid: poison ivy. Rhus toxicodendron is a wonderful remedy for arthritis, especially when the dog is very stiff upon rising but feels better after moving around for a few minutes. Rhus tox is a chilly remedy — these patients seek warm places to sleep or cuddle up.

The other major indication for Rhus tox is an ailment that comes on after a change in weather, especially when it turns cold and damp.

A combination of Rhus tox, Arnica, and Ruta graveolens is excellent for arthritis. Mix three pellets of each in a 1-ounce dropper bottle, and give one dropperful every morning.

Silicea: If you don't have Ledum on hand, or your dog was in a tussle that you didn't know about, then you may be reaching for this remedy. Silicea, made from silicon dioxide (common sand), is terrific for healing abscesses. In low potency (30C or less), it will tend to draw the abscess out and cause it to drain, getting rid of the built-up waste products of infection. Silicea is also said to help push out foreign bodies — you might want to try it for your next splinter!

Silicea patients tend to be meek, timid, sensitive, and chilly. These patients can often be characterized as "lacking grit." It is also used for vaccinosis.

Thuja: Pronounced "THOO'-yuh," this is the primary vaccinosis remedy for all species. If you must have your dog vaccinated, it is a good idea to give a dose of Thuja 30C within 2 hours of the injection. It is also helpful in case of vaccine reactions such as vomiting or diarrhea occurring within a few hours of the shot.

Thuja, which is derived from the northern white cedar, *Arbor vitae* ("Tree of Life"), is indeed a lifesaver. Thuja symptoms tend toward the skin, with rashes, eruptions, warts, cysts, and tumors being common indicators for this remedy. Its other major spheres of action are the gastrointestinal tract (it is excellent for "sputtery" diarrhea) and the urinary tract (some cases of chronic cystitis are helped by this remedy).

HOMOTOXICOLOGY

Homotoxicology was developed by German physician Hans-Heinrich Reckeweg, who broke with traditional homeopathy to establish his own line of combination remedies — remedies that contained multiple homeopathics and/or multiple potencies. Each combination, however, is proven as a single remedy just like regular homeopathics. Homotox remedies are typically low potency and broadly applicable, and homotoxicology doesn't require the precision of classical homeopathy.

In homotoxicology, we talk about something called the matrix, which is a fundamental tissue of the body. The matrix, also called ground substance, is the area in between cells. It's mostly made up of collagen and water. Blood vessels, nerves, and lymph vessels — all the tiny capillaries that make up the microcirculation — run through the matrix. Blood vessels and cells don't actually touch each other; everything has to diffuse across the matrix. Oxygen and nutrients have to diffuse into the cell, and carbon dioxide and waste products diffuse back out and get picked up by the capillaries and lymph channels. It's a very active tissue. In homotoxicology, one of the simplest but most profound concepts is that inflammation happens in the matrix.

Back in school, you may have looked at slides under the microscope; everything was pink and purple, because those were the colors of the stains used to create contrast and make everything more visible. When looking at cells, you would have seen that they have a nucleus and other little organelles like mitochondria, and that each cell is completely enclosed by a cell membrane. And surrounding the cells is some empty space containing some amorphous pink stuff, most of which is a protein called collagen; it's a sticky protein that literally holds the body together. The area between the cells where the collagen lives is called ground substance or matrix.

Whenever there's inflammation, all the white blood cells and proteins that are involved in the inflammatory reaction migrate to that area via the blood. They all gather around the tiny blood vessels — in the matrix — to prevent pathogens from getting into the cells. One consequence of this is that, with all of those immune cells and proteins in the way, nutrients and oxygen have a harder time getting to the cells, and the cells may get sick and die on account of the inflammation itself.

The body has a number of mechanisms

by which it gets rid of toxins. If you eat something bad, you'll throw it up or get diarrhea, or both. Junk in the lungs gets coughed up; harmful particles in the sinuses get sneezed out; cold and flu viruses trigger mucus production that basically floods the virus out. But if you overwhelm those normal excretory mechanisms, then the body says, "Geez, my excretory functions are already working at top speed; what will I do with the rest of this nasty stuff?" Well, if your house gets too full of stuff, what do you do? You stick it in the closet! So the matrix is like the closet (or the garage or the junk drawer); unwanted stuff gets put there to be dealt with later.

Now, we all know what happens to all that stuff in the closet — it gets neglected. In the matrix, all that debris and waste that's now sitting between the blood supply and the cells clog up the diffusion process and the cells get neglected: They don't get enough nutrients or oxygen, and waste products continue to build up in and around them.

Then what happens when you need something in the closet? If you have something in the back of the closet, you can't get to it until you take everything that's in the way out of the closet. If there is a bunch of junk between the capillaries and the cells, nothing can get across as quickly or as efficiently. Your tissues start getting toxic, and the cells start to die off. The cells are your functional tissue. For example, liver cells make things like bile and protein; kidney cells filter the blood; muscle cells contract to make the heart beat. So when too many cells die off, the whole organ becomes compromised. In most organs, when cells die, they get replaced with scar tissue. When enough cells die, that organ stops functioning. And if your vital organs aren't functioning, then you die.

Homotoxicology remedies help the body clean up the matrix. They mobilize toxins and debris to be excreted through the normal mechanisms, and they provide the right stimulus to help the organs and tissues recover. They do this gently but very efficiently. For example, the remedy Traumeel helps moderate inflammation and also stimulates the immune system to start cleaning up the tissue; the end result is healing. Muscle soreness after exertion is caused by lactic acid and cellular debris, but Traumeel mobilizes the cleanup process, and that muscle pain goes away.

FLOWER ESSENCES

Unlike potentially dangerous anti-depressants and tranquilizers, which only mask emotional distress, flower essences (sometimes called flower remedies) act as a gentle catalyst to alleviate the underlying causes of stress and to restore emotional balance. Flower essences are benign and may therefore be safely prescribed for humans, animals, and even plants. The subtlety of this therapy makes it especially well suited to the profound emotional nature of our animal companions.

Note that flower essences are not herbal remedies. Herbs possess powerful physical medicinal qualities. Herbal extracts may be made from flowers (such as chamomile and goldenseal), but flower essences are the life force collected from the energy field, or aura, of plants, without the physical properties.

The History of Flower Essences

The first formal research and development of flower essences is attributed to Dr. Edward Bach (1886–1936), a British physician, bacteriologist, and homeopath. While practicing medicine, Dr. Bach observed that his patients' state of mind was directly related to their physical ills. In 1930, he gave up his lucrative medical practice and research so he could dedicate his life to studying the relationship between the mind and the onset and progression of disease. He noticed that inharmonious states of mind, such as fear, loneliness, depression, hopelessness, and boredom, not only inhibited our natural ability to heal ourselves but also were actually the primary cause of disease itself. He believed the only way to truly cure illness was to address its underlying emotional causes, a view diametrically opposed to that of traditional medicine, which treats symptoms.

Dr. Bach ultimately developed 38 essence remedies to alleviate every negative emotional state he could identify. He also created the combination formula Rescue Remedy (Calming Essence), intended for emergency situations. Today these remedies are world renowned for their effectiveness.

No one can dispute the genius of Dr. Bach's pioneering contribution; his work has touched the lives of countless individuals and health practitioners throughout the world. Since Dr. Bach's time, many other essences have been created from flowers as well as from gems, minerals, animals, butterflies, lakes, sacred earth sites, and even stars and eclipses. Many of them are very useful in helping our animals recover from trauma, injury, and stress. These non-flower essences are often referred to as energy or vibrational essences.

How to Use Flower Essences

As you explore flower remedies, it's important to remember Dr. Bach's belief that negative thoughts and feelings poison the system, bringing about ill health and unhappiness and hindering treatment and recovery. Everyone experiences negativity from time to time, but some of us are better able to deal with it, and thus bring our systems and minds back into harmony. Flower essences help us achieve a healthful balance.

You can also include positive healing affirmations, spoken aloud when using flower remedies. We animal lovers may speak these words while administering the remedies to our animal companions. Being the highly sensitive creatures they are, they react even to subtle changes in their environment, including the moods of their human companions. Since our animal friends often suffer from the same stresses that affect us, we can take the same remedy we give our pets, saying, "I accept my feelings and deal with them openly," or whatever seems appropriate.

Especially when obvious medical problems are ruled out as the cause, flower remedies assist animals suffering from the ill effects of stress, which we know leads to disease. In fact, many behavioral problems are a sign of physical illness. Animals think; they have an active mental and emotional life. Therefore, they can similarly manifest not only behavioral but also physical problems that have their roots in emotional stress. Stress-related conditions in animals include asthma, urinary tract problems, conjunctivitis, and gastrointestinal upset (vomiting and/or diarrhea). Of course, there may be underlying physical causes for these diseases (so be sure to consult your veterinarian before assuming the cause is not medical), but acute flare-ups are very often due to emotional stress. And essences can help the animal heal the physical problems as well.

Essences heal underlying negative emotional states by "flooding" the patient with the opposite, positive quality. For example, the essence of the Bach flower remedy Holly is love. Use Holly in any situation where there is a lack of love, such as anger, jealousy, or rage. Similarly, the essence of Rock Rose is courage; it is helpful in cases of deep fears, panic, and terror.

Behavior problems such as chronic barking, obsessive-compulsive behaviors, separation anxiety, and conflicts between animals usually have a strong emotional component, so they are very treatable with essences.

Bach flower remedies may be used to complement treatment recommended by your holistic practitioner, as they seem to act as a catalyst for healing. Many homeopaths recommend their use because, unlike herbs, flower remedies don't interfere with homeopathic treatment. But other practitioners believe differently, so it's best to ask.

Administering flower remedies couldn't be easier! They can be given by mouth, in food or water, or topically. Just a few drops (3 to 5) at a time are sufficient. To increase the effect, increase the frequency rather than the volume. Add a dropperful to a spray bottle filled with spring water and use it to spray a room, carrier, kennel, or car. Or put a few drops in your hand and massage around the dog's head, ears, and paws — all of which are energy centers that will absorb the vibrations. One creative guardian, whose dog had severe separation anxiety, put a few drops on the dog's favorite stuffed toy. He was calm when she left, and was contentedly sleeping with the toy when she came home.

Since the essences act energetically, not

physically, they are completely safe and nontoxic. They cannot be overused or misused and are compatible with all other treatments. Even if you give the wrong remedy, it will not have any negative effects, but simply no effect. This allows us to use essences in food and water, even when several animals share them.

To make your own essence combination, use 2 drops of each single remedy (use 4 drops of Rescue Remedy) in a 1-ounce amber or cobalt dropper bottle filled with spring or filtered water; you may use up to 20 percent vodka in the water as a preservative (otherwise they tend to get moldy). You may use up to eight remedies, including Rescue Remedy (even though it's a combination, it counts as one when mixed with others). This will be your dosage bottle. Vigorously shake the dosage bottle against your hand to energize the remedy before administering. If you choose not to add the preservative, be sure to rinse the dropper in hot water after dosing to avoid contaminating the remainder of the formula.

In general, flower remedies are given three or four times per day. In cases of extreme stress, they may be given as often as every half hour — and Rescue Remedy may be administered every few minutes until you see improvement. If there is no improvement or symptoms worsen, seek advice from your holistic veterinarian.

When the remedies are given in food or water, there's no need to worry about their effect on your other animals. If another animal (or human, for that matter) doesn't need the remedy, it will have no effect on him, so all your animals may share the same bowls freely.

Remedy	Keynote
Agrimony	Denial, "stuffing" emotions, inappropriate communication, allergies, physical irritants
Aspen	Vague fears, sense of impending doom
Beech	Intolerance, allergies
Centaury	Meek, "doormat," picked on by other animals
Cerato	Inattentive, easily distracted
Cherry Plum	Loss of control
Chestnut Bud	To learn a lesson the first time or break habits

Chicory	Possessive, clingy, manipulative
Clematis	Consciousness, focus, after anesthesia
Crab Apple	Cleansing, infections, toxins
Elm	Easily overwhelmed or frazzled
Gentian	To see "light at the end of the tunnel," restore hope, long illness rehabilitation
Gorse	Hopelessness, giving up, cancer, critical injury or surgery
Heather	Needy, very clingy, talkative
Holly	Anger, jealousy, need for love, feeling abandoned or abused
Honeysuckle	Grief, homesickness, depleted energy
Hornbeam	Mental weariness
Impatiens	Impatience, irritability, nervous energy, pain
Larch	Lack of self-confidence

Mimulus	Timidity, specific fears, illness that does not respond to treatment
Mustard	Depression, gloom, mood swings
Oak	Chronic exhaustion, overworked but keeps struggling, loss of control
Olive	Physical exhaustion from long strain
Pine	Perfectionist, guilt, feeling rejected, abuse
Red Chestnut	Worries about others
Rescue Remedy	The five-flower combination for any acute trauma or stress. Considered as a single remedy in combination
Rock Rose	Terror, panic
Rock Water	Inflexible, stiff, arthritis
Scleranthus	Imbalance, neurologic problems
Star of Bethlehem	Trauma, need for comfort, any stray or animal from shelter

Sweet Chestnut	At wits' end, despairing
Vervain	Fanatic, hyperactive, overenthusiastic
Vine	Control, domination
Walnut	Transition, protection, oversensitive to environment
Water Violet	Grief, loner, reclusive, arrogant, to bring joy
White Chestnut	Repetitive thoughts
Wild Oat	Bored, feeling un-useful
Wild Rose	Apathy, passive resignation, to "be here now"
Willow	Resentment

Before you begin using flower remedies, look at yourself and your animal companions as objectively as possible. It's important to know which of their behaviors are normal. Many times we humans accuse animals of being spiteful or vindictive when they behave in ways we don't like, but this interpretation is often only our own inability to understand animal behavior. For instance, it's natural for puppies to bite when teething; it's not a sign of meanness or aggressiveness. But since such natural behavior isn't acceptable to us, we must find gentle ways to channel the animal's normal behavior into acceptable outlets. This way a puppy soon learns to play with toys instead.

Bach Flower Combinations for Specific Conditions

Loss of Control/Panic/Asthma Attacks*
These remedies are not a substitute for emergency medical care.

- Rescue Remedy
- Cherry Plum (anxiety attacks, incontinence, seizures, breathing difficulties)
- Rock Rose (extreme panic, breathing difficulties)
- Oak (paralysis, incontinence)

Crying, Whining, Barking
- Heather
- Beech
- Holly (especially after an interanimal conflict)
- Willow
- Agrimony

Older Pet Annoyed by Younger Animal
- Mustard
- Beech
- Wild Rose

General Irritability
- Impatiens
- Beech

History of Grief, Trauma, or Abuse
- Water Violet (grief)
- Star of Bethlehem
- Pine (guilt, animals that cringe)
- Chicory
- Honeysuckle

Boarding/Kennel/Confinement
- Heather
- Honeysuckle
- Star of Bethlehem (for comfort)
- Wild Rose
- Sweet Chestnut
- Water Violet (grief)
- Wild Oat (boredom)

Separation Anxiety
- Chicory
- Wild Oat
- Holly
- Willow
- Wild Rose
- Heather

Conflicts among Animals
- Willow (resentment)
- Agrimony (open communication and harmony)
- Mimulus (for picked-on animal)
- Vine (for dominant, bully animal)
- Beech
- Holly
- Walnut

Training Formula
- Clematis
- Chestnut Bud
- Cerato

Travel Remedy
(* = 3 remedies that make up the Basic Formula)

- Rescue Remedy★
- Elm★
- Walnut★
- Mimulus (fear of riding in car)
- Cherry Plum (for panic in car)
- Scleranthus (for car sickness, balance problems)

Recovery Assistance

- Gentian (to give hope)
- Gorse (for animals who have "given up")
- Centaury (increases the will to live)
- Sweet Chestnut (for increased energy)
- Olive (for physical exhaustion)
- Honeysuckle (restores depleted energy)

When you consider that every animal is an individual made of the same "stuff" we are, it isn't any wonder that by observing their personalities and traits, we can prescribe flower essences and blends for them as easily as we can for ourselves and our whole family.

EMOTIONAL FREEDOM TECHNIQUES (TAPPING)

The Emotional Freedom Techniques (EFT) therapy, or "Tapping," is one of the most amazing healing modalities ever discovered. It's free to learn and easy to apply. We recommend it for both people and animals, especially together!

Let's take a look at how EFT works in people, which we hope will encourage you to learn and apply it in everyday situations as well as for chronic physical and emotional issues. If we are emotionally and physically healthier, we will naturally be better parents to our Paleo Dogs, as well as get more joy out of life ourselves!

We all have certain habits of thought and patterns of behavior that hinder us from being all we can be and from doing all we can do. In our experience, many animal lovers, especially those involved in rescue, trap-neuter-return, etc., have a huge heart for animals but never enough money. How much more could we help animals if we could only break through our own financially limiting beliefs! Lots of programs make great claims about instant wealth and happiness, but as they say, "If it seems too good to be true, it probably is." EFT, however, is the one modality that really can cut to the core of any issue and can truly resolve deeply buried conflicts and emotions that are hiding behind the scenes, running the show.

EFT is a method of tapping certain points along traditional Chinese acupuncture meridians to resolve emotional, behavioral, and physical problems. It is one of the new schools of meridian energy therapies and was developed by Gary Craig, who studied thought field therapy (TFT), the first of many tapping therapies. By tapping on these points while keeping a specific problem in mind, negative energy is cleared, often in a rapid and dramatic way.

EFT is easily adapted to remote or proxy (surrogate) use, and the technique can be learned in a few minutes. First bring to mind the problem. If it is a large or deep-seated problem, such as a phobia, it is best to focus on one specific aspect of the problem at a time. Instead of a general or large (global) issue like soiling in the house, consider a specific one such as "Spot urinates under the table." Think of the problem as a forest: To get rid of the forest, you have to remove individual trees one at a time. Minor problems can often be cleared up with one or two rounds of tapping.

Using EFT on dogs is especially easy — you don't even need to tap on the dog. While animals do have meridians and points, the best way to perform EFT on animals is by surrogate or proxy tapping. This means you tap on yourself to make the changes happen.

How to Perform EFT

Note: It is helpful to drink a glass of spring water before you begin your EFT session and to take three deep cleansing breaths.

1. First, think of a phrase or a sentence that describes the problem succinctly and clearly to you. You can say, "Sidney keeps licking his right front paw," or "Sam keeps pestering me while I'm cooking dinner." Begin by saying, "Even though [insert the name of your dog]" and then say the problem as a statement, and follow with the positive phrase, "I deeply and profoundly love and accept [insert dog's name]." This is your opening statement.
2. Find the "Karate Chop Point," which is the place on the side of your hand that, if you were a karate master, you would use to smash a 2 × 4 or cinder block. You can use either hand; tap on that spot with the fingers of the opposite hand.
3. Repeat the opening statement three times while continuously tapping the Karate Chop Point.
4. Now choose a shortened version of the opening statement, called the "reminder phrase." Tap with one or two fingers 5 to 10 times on the following spots (either side is fine) as you say the reminder statement

395

once on each point.

Eyebrow: Where the bone behind your eyebrow meets the bridge of your nose

Corner of the eye: On the bone at the outside corner of your eye

Under the eye: On the bone just below your eye, in line with your pupil if you look straight ahead

Under the nose: Between your nose and your upper lip

Chin: In the indentation between your chin and your lower lip

Underarm: In line with a man's nipples on the side of the body; somewhat lower and toward the back for a woman

Collarbone: In the angle formed by your collarbone and the breastbone

Crown: Pat the crown of your head with your flat open hand

5. When you're finished with each round, inhale and exhale deeply.

EFT TAPPING POINTS

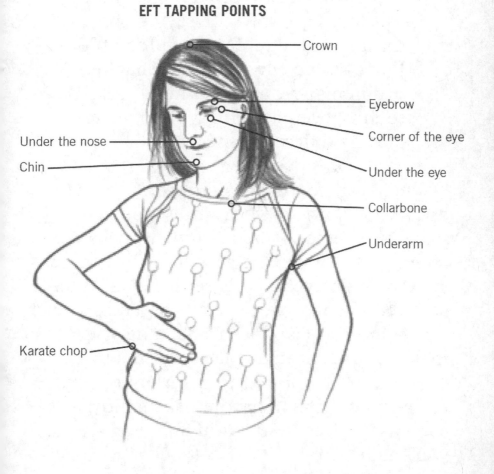

Crown

Eyebrow

Corner of the eye

Under the nose

Under the eye

Chin

Collarbone

Underarm

Karate chop

You can repeat the treatment with different statements. Your intuition will often suggest new phrases as you do this. Different statements create different changes, so experiment with many different forms of wording and ways of saying something until you feel comfortable. For chronic physical or behavioral problems, you may need many rounds over a period of time, exploring different aspects.

When you focus your attention on your dog, you connect your individual energy systems together. When you then focus your attention on a specific aspect of that energy system (a problem, disease, behavior, etc.), and you change your system by tapping on the points, you are also changing the animal's system through that connection.

EFT can be applied to a variety of physical and emotional problems, including issues associated with aging. For example, you might work with the following aspects for a dog who soils inside the house:

- "Even though Spot feels a need to do his business in the house, I deeply and completely love and accept him."

- "Even though Spot feels his territory is being threatened . . ."
- "Even though Spot doesn't get along with Muffy the cat . . ."
- "Even though I get upset when Spot soils in the house . . ." (This and similar aspects address the guardian's emotional issues, which can be a significant part of the problem!)

As you go along, other phrases may suggest themselves to you; keep tapping on each additional aspect that comes up. Allow your intuition to guide you.

Try EFT for everything: allergies, asthma, conflicts, past traumas, pain, and all kinds of disease. (See "Professional Specialists" in Resources for contact information to learn more about EFT.)

Once you feel that you have cleared everything you can in one session, take three deep cleansing breaths and drink a glass of water.

NAMBUDRIPAD'S ALLERGY ELIMINATION TECHNIQUE

Nambudripad's Allergy Elimination Technique (NAET) is a diagnostic and treatment technique based on the principles of Chinese medicine and acupuncture. It was developed for humans by Devi Nambudripad, DC, PhD, LAc, RN. Veterinarians have extended the use of NAET to domestic pets. NAET can be performed in the vet's office or over the phone. Factors that contribute to premature aging, such as emotional trauma and other stressors, can be offset with the use of NAET because it is so effective at calming the immune system and reducing inflammation.

Allergies are one of the most common problems that pets face today. While, strictly speaking, an allergy is a very specific type of immune reaction, usually to a protein, in NAET, allergies are considered to be an unusual sensitivity to any substance. Allergies may result from repeated exposure to an allergen over a long period of time (food allergies are a common example), brief exposure to a very strong or toxic substance, or from events such as serious trauma, major surgery, and vaccination.

NAET offers an energy-medicine solution to allergic conditions. Muscle testing such as applied kinesiology is used to confirm the presence of allergic reactivity. Once the allergy is identified, acupuncture and/or acupressure is used to eliminate it by reprogramming the body's response to future contact. A specific protocol has been developed that prioritizes treatment of common as well as unique allergens. NAET training is only available to professionals. (See Resources on page 527.)

TESLA'S PURPLE PLATES

Purple or "positive energy" plates are based on legendary physicist Nikola Tesla's theories about energy or the etheric medium that fills all of space and from which all matter originates. Of course, Albert Einstein proved the equivalence of energy and matter with his equation $E = mc^2$, and Tesla's etheric energy is now called dark matter by physicists worldwide. Tesla worked with Thomas Edison for many years and contributed to the development of the alternating current we depend on today, as well as radio transmission and much more. His name is designated as the unit of measurement for magnetic field strength.

An inventor named Ralph Bergstresser worked on the theory behind the purple plates with Tesla for 20 years. After Tesla's death, Bergstresser finally created them by altering the atomic structure in aluminum plates so that they generate a positive energy field around them. This energy is said to penetrate anything placed on or near it.

Advocates of the plates believe that this

energy benefits plants, people, and pets. The plates are thought to hasten healing, raise energy levels, and protect against electromagnetic fields.

You can place purple plates under your dog's bed, food, or water dishes, or attach a disk to your dog's collar. You can also put purple disks on your cell phone and computer to limit harmful electromagnetic fields. Many people use purple plates under produce to keep it fresh longer. (See Resources on page 534.)

CRYSTALS

Crystals are created when water combines with a mineral element under certain conditions of pressure, temperature, and energy. Crystals don't interact directly with the physical body but rather with the fundamental energy system that creates and supports the body, and connects it with the mind and emotions. The physical body exists only by virtue of energy; we get energy from food, water, air, and the earth itself. In conjunction with the mind, crystals can create all types of healing that manifest in the physical body.

Crystals pick up the energies of the people and places where they have been, and they accumulate both positive and negative vibrations. Negative energies can also come from electromagnetic radiation from televisions, cell phones, and computers.

When you first acquire crystals, you should always cleanse them as soon as you can. Here are a few possibilities.

- Smudge the crystals with sage and sweetgrass or your favorite incense by passing the crystal through the smoke several times.
- Rinse the crystals in running water. Check first to make sure that your type of crystal can tolerate water.
- Set your crystal in or on sea salt or Himalayan salt. Check first to make sure that your type of crystal can tolerate salt.
- Set your crystal in or on a large quartz crystal, citrine, or amethyst cluster.
- Cleanse your crystal with flower essences or Reiki.
- When the crystals are cleansed, fill them with your positive intentions to keep them from reabsorbing negative energy. Recleanse them after use.

Tumbled or polished stones seem to open up and increase energy and may easily be used under seat cushions, dog beds, and birthing beds; or place one in the water bowl to energize your pet's purified water.

As mentioned above, crystals can be used very effectively with color therapy and chakra energy healing.

ACUPUNCTURE/ACUPRESSURE

Acupuncture is a technique that stimulates specific points in the body to rectify energy imbalances. According to legend, thousands of years ago someone noticed that lame warhorses, when wounded by arrows in certain spots, would stop limping. (Another legend tells a similar tale about humans.) The same spots were stimulated in other lame horses, who also stopped limping.

After the energy pathways of the body were discovered and mapped, it was concluded that any disruption of the energy flow, qi (or chi), caused disease. Placing small needles along exact points on these energy pathways was found to enhance the flow of qi and promote a state of health. Today acupuncturists may choose from among metal needles, heat, pressure, massage, electrical stimulation, injections, magnets, gold beads, lasers, or any combination of these.

Human and veterinary acupuncture began separately, using different charts because the pathways (meridians and collaterals) are somewhat different in a four-legged animal than in an upright human.

Impressed by research and clinical results, the American Veterinary Medical Association sanctioned further study of acupuncture as a valid method of treatment in 1989. Many holistic veterinarians now embrace this technique in their practices. To become certified, a veterinarian must complete a 4-month-long training course accredited by the International Veterinary Acupuncture Society (see Resources on page 511), pass an oral and a written exam, and submit a complete report of a successful acupuncture case.

Acupuncture for Your Dog

Animal acupuncture is used to treat arthritis, spinal and disk problems, kidney disorders, metabolic imbalances, aging disorders, cataracts, asthma, and allergic dermatitis. It can be helpful in unblocking obstructed urethras in unneutered males and may be used during surgical emergencies for shock and respiratory arrest, to treat infertility, and to build immune response. Have your acupuncturist show you how to needle the emergency rescue point; nonbreathing puppies and kittens can sometimes be resuscitated this way.

Relief of ailments often comes after only one acupuncture treatment, but it usually takes at least three visits before dramatic results are seen. The most difficult thing about acupuncture is that some animals may get worse before they get better. But once they weather the crisis, their improvement may be quite dramatic and enduring.

Acupuncture is especially effective for musculoskeletal problems, such as hip dysplasia and arthritis, and for problems involving nerves or the spinal cord. However, in the hands of a skilled practitioner, internal issues and even behavioral problems can be addressed. Acupuncture is also very helpful in postoperative care.

Most often, acupuncture involves inserting needles into the acupuncture points. The needles used in acupuncture are smaller in diameter than those used to give injections. Once in place, they are not painful, and most animals relax or even fall asleep during treatment. Other methods may also be used — which can be troublesome for some animals — including electrically stimulating a point, injecting a solution into a point, heating a point, applying finger pressure to or massaging the point, and implanting gold beads or seeds at a

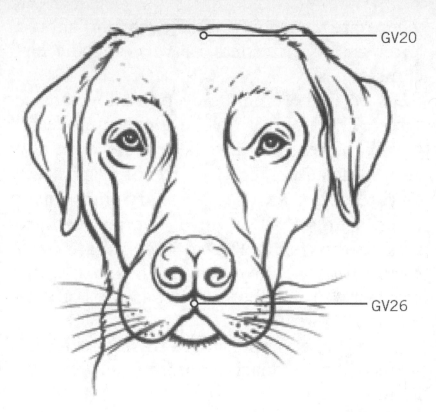

GV20

GV26

point (this can also be done under an anesthetic).

Acupressure Treatments for Your Dog

While acupuncture therapy should be left to a qualified practitioner, acupressure is a technique you can learn and do at home.

To perform acupressure on a specific point, use the tip of your index finger or thumb to press firmly but gently. (If you get a "flinching" reaction, or the animal cries out, you're probably pressing too hard!)

There are two points that everyone should know that are needed for very specific circumstances.

GV 26 is the emergency point for cardiac arrest. This point is on the Governing Vessel meridian, centered just below the nose and above the upper lip. In case of respiratory or cardiac arrest, use any sharp instrument (even a fingernail) to give a series of sharp jabs to this point. You may stimulate newborn pups if they are having difficulty breathing or, for that matter, are not breathing at all.

However, never stimulate this point in this manner on a conscious animal, or you risk getting bitten!

GV 20 is also on the Governing Vessel meridian. It is the master point for energy and emotional balance. Whether your dog is lethargic or hyperactive, dominant or shy, depressed or manic, GV 20 is a great point to return your dog's energy to perfect balance.

Association Points

Association points run along the Bladder Meridian, on the dog's back along the muscles on either side of the spine. The association points correspond to each specific organ meridian. Run your fingers slowly

408

along this pair of meridians, with firm but gentle pressure. Note if and where your dog tenses or flinches; this may indicate an imbalance in the associated organ or system. Sensitivity to light pressure may signal an acute condition, whereas the dog may be more tender to deep pressure where there is chronic disease. (See Resources on page 511.)

TRADITIONAL CHINESE MEDICINE — CIRCADIAN CLOCK

There are 12 meridians (energy pathways) in the body that are linked to 12 specific organs. In traditional Chinese medicine, each organ has a 2-hour time period when the qi (life energy) is at its peak in that meridian. Here is a diagram of the times and organ systems in the Chinese clock.

Pay attention to symptoms that occur repeatedly at specific times, because this may indicate that an organ is out of balance; having this information will be helpful to your holistic veterinarian.

ENERGY MEDICINE DEVICES

Many devices target the energetic fields in and around us to neutralize damaging radiation and support healing in the body. These can also be considered antiaging since they

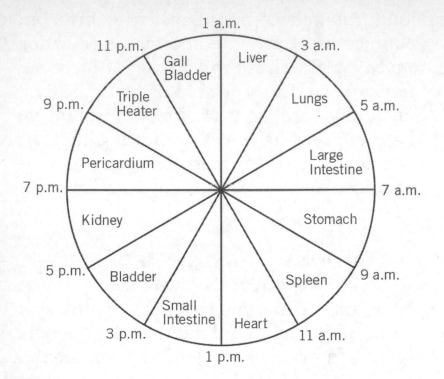

purport to prevent oxidative cellular damage as well as heal that which is already present. There is less hard science supporting many of these devices, yet thousands of compelling reports from people who have experienced healing for themselves and their pets are hard to ignore. In this section, we provide an overview of the field of energy healing, and we suggest that you discuss the most appropriate therapies for your dog with your holistic veterinarian.

The basic concept behind energy medicine is that all life-forms are submerged in the electromagnetic field of Earth. Additionally, each life-form has its own electromagnetic field that, when distorted enough, results in disease. Earth's electromagnetic field provides the link between the practitioner and patient during analysis and treatment. It is an ancient axiom that energy follows thought, and thought is transmitted through the energy field of Earth, allowing the practitioner to attune himself to the patient.

The BEMER System

The BEMER (Bio-Electro-Magnetic-Energy Regulation) system is a thoroughly researched, patented, FDA-registered Class I medical device. The core of BEMER technology is a multidimensional wave signal that stimulates impaired microcirculation. Defective microcirculation underlies health complaints and illnesses; it is also a major factor in the degenerative changes that occur over time — in other words, aging. Consistent use of BEMER technology is a wonderful adjunct to holistic and conventional care. Among its benefits are the following:

- Improved supply and waste disposal for organs and tissue

- Support for healing wounds and injuries
- Immune system support

The BEMER technology supports all regeneration processes in the organism. This results in a wide range of complementary applications for numerous conditions. The BEMER system can be used at home, and doctors and veterinarians are using the BEMER technology in their clinics with great success. (See Resources on page 511.)

The NanoVi Device

Repairing damage from free radicals is a normal cellular activity. Problems arise only when the repair is not sufficient to counteract the damage. The NanoVi bio-identical signaling technology can be used to help the body boost these repair activities.

The NanoVi and the NanoVi Pro devices work in the same way, but the Pro device is more powerful, so it takes less time for a session. When considering whether a particular protocol is right for you and your human and animal family, you can always look into the testing that has been conducted. Measures of oxidative stress damage and DNA repair are good ways of validating this particular approach. (See Resources on page 511.)

Bioresonance Therapies

As quantum physics proves, matter and energy are one and the same; this is the meaning of Einstein's great equation $E = mc^2$. As a result, we can influence physical matter by altering its energy fields. Bioresonance, also called bio-energetics, is the field of frequency therapy that seeks to bring energy fields into harmony or resonance.

Bioresonance instruments are intended to detect and correct pathological dysfunctions in people, plants, and animals before any physical conditions or symptoms arise. It's obviously better to catch problems early before pathology is established in the body!

There are hundreds of bioresonance techniques and instruments.

Radionics, one of the most durable therapies, went "underground" because of persecution by the FDA and other government agencies, but it remains popular. There is a "virtual" radionics instrument called the SE05, or "paper training model," that is thought to produce the same results as a radionics machine, making it available to anyone. The Sai Sanjeevini system is a cross between radionics and flower essences; it's

413

very safe and is freely accessible online (see Resources on page 511).

Other bioresonance therapies include Electrodermal Screening (EDS), Rife therapy, Intrinsic Data Fields, CoRe, Quantum Xeroid Consciousness Interface (QXCI), Ondamed, Scientific Consciousness Interface Operations System (SCIO), Life-System, Bicom, Nutri-Energetics Systems (NES), Self-Controlled Energo Neuro Adaptive Regulation (SCENAR), Vega Testing, Wave Maker, Chi Machine, and Vibrational Integrated Bio-photonic Energizer (VIBE) Machine.

Veterinarians in the future, using one or more of these devices, and properly trained in these technologies, may be able to recognize potential danger signs and pinpoint and eliminate disease-producing toxins from the body long before they can become destructive. Perhaps one day we'll look back on invasive treatments such as drugs, vaccinations, and surgery as if they were techniques of the Dark Ages. Until then, our best alternative is to stay abreast of developments in human regenerative medicine. The more demand for wellness, life extension, and antiaging breakthroughs, the more our veterinarians will study these subjects and provide this care to our dogs.

We suggest caution, careful research, and training before relying on any of these devices for a diagnosis or treatment. Always consult your veterinarian before implementing any of these energy modalities.

AFTERWORD

As we look toward the future, we see two potential paths for canine-kind. The first is the road we seem to be most determined to travel. This road leads to more and more technology, more refined medical interventions, and more usurping of our own common sense by the pet food industry. This is really the Path of Profit, in which the nature and needs of our dogs are subsumed by a culture of greed.

The other path goes along the edges of the first before emerging in new hope as more and more people learn about natural, holistic options for their dogs as well as themselves. On this path, we will turn away from individual and environmental destruction and massive profit margins and move toward a sustainable future where the whole is the prime consideration, whether the whole person, whole dog, or whole planet.

If we look beyond what we have been

taught about "evidenced-based medicine," we can ponder the possibility of a world where we might never again need a physician or a veterinarian.

What if we *did* know how to not only heal ourselves but also to prevent disease? What if *all* healing could be done inside our own minds, which could then be extended to our family and companion animals? We believe that we already have this ability, but we just don't have the confidence or the know-how to implement it.

Our future can be consciously empowered with the knowledge that if we can get ourselves into a particular state of health, we also have the power to get ourselves out of it. We might be able to heal ourselves and our dogs by understanding the true power of these belief systems and implementing them with confidence and love.

APPENDIX A: SUPPLEMENTS

Caution: Do not experiment with supplements, especially if your dog has a medical condition. Get safe dosages designed for your dog from a veterinarian well versed in clinical nutrition. Always avoid products containing any form of sugar or artificial sweetener, especially xylitol (which is toxic to dogs), or sodium benzoate (a preservative).

SUPPLEMENTS FOR PALEO DOG RECIPES

There are a number of products made to supplement homemade pet diets. This is an ever-changing market, but we assessed the products available as we were writing this book.

Balance IT Carnivore Blend is a veterinarian-formulated vitamin and mineral powder containing a full array of AAFCO-specified nutrients, but many are

We prefer "whole food supplements" because when you isolate a vitamin, a mineral, or another nutrient out of its natural food complex, where it is an inseparable part of a vast web of known and unknown factors such as enzymes, protein chaperones, phytonutrients, etc., it is no longer beneficial to life. This is especially true in the case of vertebrate mammals, who are designed to get their nutrients from the plants they ingest, from the prey who ingested plants, or through the biotransformation of inorganic minerals to organic ones by microflora in their gastrointestinal tracts.

A whole food source of a mineral will often recommend a lower nutrient dose on the label than a chemical compound or an isolate. This does not mean that the whole food product is less potent. On the contrary, it means that the food-based supplement is so bioavailable that you don't have to use as much. The results are better and longer lasting. To truly go Paleo, we don't use supplements the way that drugs are used, to palliate or suppress symptoms. We want to nourish the dog's body so that it operates optimally and can continue to maintain, repair, and heal itself.

synthetic and not derived from whole foods.

Canine Vitamin and Mineral Mixture, available at MyPetGrocer.com, is recommended for cooked homemade diets; it uses synthetic vitamins.

Fresh + Oasis Canine is a "just add meat" supplement. It claims to be complete but does not include a source of omega-3 fatty acids, and it guarantees only 13 out of the 36 AAFCO-required nutrients. It appears to contain some synthetic ingredients, but on the plus side, many of the minerals are chelated (a more absorbable and usable form) and it contains probiotics. It also contains yeast and dairy products, which are a common allergen in dogs.

Furoshnikov's Formulas claim to make a complete and balanced diet when added to meat, but they contain only synthetic vitamins.

Grandma Lucy's Artisan and Performance premixes are intended to be added to meat, but they contain a lot of carbohydrates as well as synthetic vitamins. They provide an AAFCO-compliant diet when added to meat.

Natural Diet Foundation 2, developed by Wendy Volhard, is largely made from whole foods, but oats is the top ingredient.

Sojos Original Dog Food Mix and Grain-

Free Dog Food Mix are intended to be added to meat to make a complete diet but are loaded with carbohydrates.

Urban Wolf claims to meet or exceed AAFCO requirements, but the calcium-to-phosphorus ratio appears to be too high. It contains potatoes and other carbohydrates as well as yeast.

Centrum, the human product, is recommended by many veterinary nutritionists for dogs on a homemade diet. Clearly, they have never read the label, because Centrum provides only a fraction of most vitamins and minerals. We do not consider it suitable for people, let alone pets.

Recommended Products

Celestial Pets: Unlike other "just add meat" products, Celestial Pets is a three-product set that includes a vitamin-mineral mix, an essential fatty acid oil blend, and an enzyme blend. It is made exclusively from whole foods and has a stellar 20-plus-year track record with thousands of pets. All ingredients are US-sourced only.

- **Celestial Pets VitaMineral Plus** is a vitamin-mineral premix made for a homemade raw-meat diet that contains organic bone meal from New Zealand, glandular extracts, super greens concentrate, and other whole food supplements.

- **Celestial Pets Essential Fatty Acid Oil** is an essential fatty acid supplement containing omega-3s, omega-6s, and omega-9s.
- **Celestial Pets Enzyme Supplement** is a complete enzyme supplement containing fungal-source protease, lipase, amylase, and cellulase, as well as probiotics, vacuum-dried liver, and pancreas extract.

Moxxor is a proprietary blend of essential fatty acids including 18 unique forms of powerful anti-inflammatory marine lipids and potent antioxidants from New Zealand green-lipped mussel oil, its primary ingredient. This cold-extracted oil is naturally preserved with super-antioxidants from organic sauvignon blanc grape seed husk extract and kiwifruit seed oil, which contains all eight natural forms of vitamin E. No filler oils or excipients are used in Moxxor.

PROBIOTICS

The term *probiotics* (which means "promoting life") covers a variety of "friendly" bacteria that are beneficial for the digestive tract. These include *Lactobacillus acidophilus* and other *Lactobacillus* species and certain strains of *Bacillus, Enterococcus, Bifidobacteria,* and *Streptococcus,* all of which are commonly found in over-the-counter probiotic supplements.

Probiotics are of special importance in dogs with any type of digestive problem, including vomiting, diarrhea, and constipation. They are essential for animals who are, or have been, taking antibiotics; they can be given both during the course of antibiotics and for at least 2 weeks afterward. Probiotics are particularly useful for allergies, including atopy (inhalant allergies), food allergies, and inflammatory bowel disease.

Probiotics promote a balanced and healthy bacterial population in the gut, which is important for complete digestion and general well-being. Intestinal bacteria aid in digesting certain nutrients by providing enzymes that the body does not make on its own. These organisms manufacture several B vitamins and help maintain proper pH in the gut. They also prevent colonization of the digestive tract by pathological (disease-causing) organisms such as *Salmonella.*

Probiotic bacteria are normally present in a healthy digestive tract, mainly in the colon. *L. acidophilus,* the strain most often used in fermented products such as yogurt, was the first to be isolated and used as therapy, initially to treat constipation and diarrhea in human patients in the 1920s and '30s. In one study, human patients were given antibiotics to kill off most of their normal gut flora. After the antibiotic course was finished, they were given *L. acidophilus* supplements. Interestingly, the levels of other normal bacteria, such as *Enterococci,* also normalized rapidly. Further studies showed that the probiotics must be taken daily to maintain the beneficial effects.

More recent research on probiotics has found that few, if any, commercial probiotic supplements made for pets actually contain live bacteria, despite label claims to the contrary. That doesn't sound like good news, but it turns out that even these "dead" bacteria have a clear and beneficial impact on digestion. It seems that even after they've given up the ghost, probiotic bacteria still provide nutrients and other immune-boosting factors that help the intestinal cells stay healthy and happy.

It's easy to add probiotics to your dog's diet. While many owners and breeders recommend adding a tablespoon of yogurt to the food, this does not contain enough organisms to have any significant effect.

Most yogurt made with live cultures contains *L. acidophilus* and similar organisms at much lower levels, in the neighborhood of 100,000 colony-forming units per milliliter (CFU/ml). It is better and simpler (and definitely more cost-effective) to buy human-grade probiotics in powder or capsules and add them to the food. Choose a probiotic supplement that contains at least *Lactobacillus* and *Bifidobacteria*. Many probiotics must be kept refrigerated to keep the organisms viable. Fortunately, these supplements generally have little taste and are readily accepted by most pets if mixed with food.

DIGESTIVE ENZYMES

Enzymes are the workhorses that perform virtually every function in the body. There are thousands of enzymes in every living cell, some of which are digestive enzymes (also called lysozymes).

The dog's natural diet of raw prey takes advantage of the natural enzymes in the prey's body to aid in digestion. Cooking and processing of food destroys (denatures) these vital enzymes. Without them, the dog's pancreas must secrete more digestive enzymes to compensate. Such artificially created stress is a precursor to a great number

of chronic and acute health proble
(Cooking also reduces the water con
and alters the protein structure of the meat,
making it more difficult to digest.)

A balanced enzyme product (containing
protease for protein, lipase for fats, and if
you're feeding veggies, amylase to digest
carbohydrates and cellulase to break down
plant cell walls) must always be added to
any cooked or processed dog food product
to help the dog digest the food thoroughly
and get the maximum benefit from the nutrients.

Enzymes are also used with the raw homemade diet as well, especially if raw vegetables are included. This is because, in the
wild, the dog would obtain this vegetable
matter predigested in the prey animals' gastrointestinal tract, where digestive enzymes
would have already done their job.

We recommend a formula created by a
holistic veterinarian: Celestial Pets Digestive Enzymes. Simply follow the amounts
recommended on the label. Digestive enzymes are of critical importance and especially so when making any change to your
dog's diet.

OMEGA-3 FATTY ACIDS

The omegas are simply different types of fat molecules. Despite all the low-fat hype we see every day from advertisers, fats are vital elements of your dog's diet. The body uses them to build cell walls, to manufacture hormones, to protect brain cells, and for thousands of other functions.

Fatty acids are specific types of polyunsaturated fats. These fats are liquid at room temperature because they contain one or more double bonds that put a "kink" in the long, thin molecules, preventing them from packing together closely. Saturated fat molecules, on the other hand, have no double bonds and can bunch up close together, like teenagers in a mosh pit. This makes them solid at room temperature.

The two main classes of essential fatty acids are the omega-3s and the omega-6s. They are called essential because the body (human or canine) cannot make them; they must be obtained in the diet.

(Warning: Science ahead! Skip this paragraph if you hated high school chemistry!) The number after "omega" indicates where the last double bond is located: either 3 or 6 carbons from the end of the chain (Omega is the last letter of the Greek alphabet). There are other classes of fatty acids, such as omega-7 (found in macadamia nuts, green-lipped mussels, and sea buckthorn) and omega-9 (found in olive oil, avocados, and some nuts), but they are not considered essential. There is a specific method to naming them. For example, linoleic acid, found in grape seed oil, is designated "18:2n6," where 18 is the number of carbons in the chain, there are 2 double-bonds, and it is an omega-6.

Omega-3 fatty acids are said to be anti-inflammatory and omega-6's pro-inflammatory because of the way they are used in the body to make certain hormones; one pathway suppresses, and the other promotes inflammation.

Our dogs' natural diet — wild prey — contains plenty of omega-3s, as does livestock's natural diet of grass. However, commercial pet foods are universally deficient in high-quality omega-3 fatty acids because of the way livestock and poultry are raised in the United States and Canada. Their corn-based diet reduces their natural omega-3 content by almost 90 percent and shifts the fatty acid balance to nearly all omega-6.[1] Unfortunately, this goes for nearly all the meat you can buy at the grocery store; even organic and natural meats have the same problem. Only organic

percent grass-fed meat and 100 percent
ıre-raised poultry and eggs provide the
natural fatty acid balance that our dogs
need.

The omega fatty acids are important for
healthy skin. Often, the first sign of an
imbalance or deficiency shows up as dry,
dull fur or itchy, irritated, or flaky skin. Both
omega-3s and omega-6s are helpful in such
cases.

Omega-3s, in particular, perform many
vital functions: They help maintain flexible
cell membranes, keep the skin healthy, and
are used to produce many vital hormones
and other compounds. Omega-3s also have
strong anti-inflammatory properties. Inflammation is involved in the development of
many chronic diseases, including allergies,
arthritis, autoimmune disease, and many
gastrointestinal diseases. Omega-3s help our
pets resist age-related and degenerative
conditions such as arthritis,[2] asthma,[3]
chronic renal failure,[4] obesity,[5] heart disease,[6] cancer,[7] age-related cognitive dysfunction (senility),[8] and even behavioral issues such as aggression.[9]

There are many sources of omega-3s out
there, and each makes its own fabulous
claims. We've not only thoroughly researched these sources, but we've also tried

them for ourselves and our pets. Our conclusions surprised even us!

Flaxseed/Nuts/Vegetable Oils

The vast majority of plant-based oils (such as corn, safflower, sunflower, soybean, canola, and peanut) are omega-6 fatty acids, which are already vastly oversupplied in our pets' diets. However, flaxseeds and a few other seeds and nuts also contain an omega-3 called alpha-linolenic acid (ALA). Unfortunately, dogs cannot convert more than 1 to 2 percent of it into eicosapentaenoic acid (EPA) and docosahexaenoic acid (DHA) — the essential forms that are so important for our pets. The only forms of the most important omega-3s that are bio-available to our pets must be obtained from an animal source, such as marine lipids. (Note: Always give extra vitamin E when supplementing with oils that do not already contain it.)

Fish-Based Oils

Fish oils and cod-liver oil are the most common and popular sources of EPA and DHA. However, these are surprisingly problematic.

Most salmon oil (and all salmon products from the Atlantic Ocean, Scotland, and Norway) comes from farm-raised salmon.

These fish are grown in polluted, over-crowded pens; they are heavily vaccinated and fed antifungals, parasiticides, and antibiotics; and they contain up to 10 times more mercury, dioxins, PCBs, and other toxins than wild fish.[10] They contain far more omega-6s than does wild salmon. Farmed salmon also pose a serious threat to wild species in both the Atlantic and Pacific Oceans from disease and interbreeding of escaped fish. Additionally, about one-third of salmon that are labeled "Alaska," "wild," or "wild-caught" are not truly wild, but rather bred and raised in hatcheries.[11] Their release to the ocean is threatening both wild salmon and other fish.[12]

Cod-liver oil is commonly supplemented with vitamins A and D, at levels that could easily become toxic in small dogs. Moreover, a loophole in the law allows non-cod species (such as whitefish, pollock, and scrod) to be labeled as cod.

Oils made from other fish, such as sardine, herring, and anchovy oils, are — so far — more sustainable and cleaner than most other fish oils. However, a small fish called menhaden is the source of most unspecified "fish oil." Menhaden is heavily harvested for many purposes. Unfortunately, it is a threatened keystone species, so menhaden

products should be avoided for enviror
tal and sustainability reasons.[13]

Krill oil is a non-fish alternative omega-ɔ
product that is gaining in popularity. Krill
(tiny red shrimplike crustaceans) are the
major food source for many marine animals,
including fish, whales, seals, squid, and
birds. Krill are utilized for oil as well as being processed into food for farmed fish. The
global biomass of krill is enormous, but the
problem is that they are being harvested
near critical feeding grounds of the animals
that eat them, potentially threatening dozens
of species, from fish to seabirds to whales.[14]

New Zealand green-lipped mussels (*Perna
canaliculus*) are grown in a sustainable
farming program that ensures the long-term
viability of the mussel population as well as
minimum impact on the environment.
Green-lipped mussels are bivalve mollusks
that are a rich source of 33 fatty acids,
including 18 omega-3s (among them EPA,
DHA, and ALA). One of the green-lipped
mussels' unique array of omega-3s is ETA
(eicosatetraenoic acid), which is not found
in any other foods to any measurable degree
and which has extremely powerful anti-
inflammatory properties.[15] We recommend
Moxxor (see above), as the best-quality
green-lipped mussel oil supplement.

ANTIOXIDANTS:
THE ANTIAGING SUPPLEMENTS

Antioxidants are natural compounds that are important in the neutralization or scavenging of oxygen free radicals, which are normal by-products of body metabolism. Controlled amounts of free radicals are made by the body as weapons against viruses and bacteria and are used in hormone production and numerous cellular reactions.

However, excess free radicals can damage cellular DNA, destroy cell membranes, and lead to chronic inflammation, degenerative diseases, immune system damage, and even cancer.

Excessive amounts of free radicals can result from exposure to radiation, including sunlight, and environmental pollution and from an unhealthy diet. In people, a diet high in fresh fruits and vegetables may contain adequate natural antioxidants. Pets eating commercial food, however, do not get enough appropriate antioxidants in the diet; and even pets eating a perfect Paleo Diet can always use a little extra support in this toxic world.

There are many good antioxidant supplements. Where dosage information isn't specified, give a small dog between 1/10 to

1/6 of the human dosage, as specified on the label, per day. A human dose is calculated for a 150-pound person, so dosages should be adjusted for larger dogs by their weight. (But do not exceed the human dose no matter how big your dog is.) Using multiple antioxidants in combination is more effective than large doses of single products. Please consult your holistic veterinarian for specific product and dosage recommendations.

Here are some antioxidants that may be helpful in pets.

Vitamin C is a powerful antioxidant and has many other important functions. Dogs can produce their own vitamin C, but in an amount that is likely insufficient to meet the challenges of modern life discussed in Chapter 5. Avoid supplements that contain only synthetic ascorbic acid made from corn; use sodium ascorbate, calcium ascorbate, or Ester-C. Vitamin C may be dosed to "bowel tolerance." That is, you start off adding just a little vitamin C (25 to 50 milligrams) to the food and increase the dose very gradually until diarrhea develops. At that point, go back to the previous dosage amount that did not cause diarrhea and stay with that dose. Note that an individual pet's tolerance may vary, depending on diet, time of year, and stress level. In general, 100 milligrams per day is plenty for a small dog, 500 milligrams for a large dog.

Vitamin E in its natural form is d-alpha-tocopherol. Avoid synthetic vitamin E (dl-alpha-tocopherol). If the label says just "alpha," it's probably the synthetic (cheaper) kind. While alpha-tocopherols are more common, a product containing "mixed" tocopherols and trienols (there are eight of them) may have more benefits. A small dog may take 100 IU per day, and a very large dog up to 400 IU per day.

Proanthocyanidins (pycnogenol/pine bark extract and grape seed extract) are highly concentrated antioxidants that are easy and fairly inexpensive to use.

Chlorophyll, the plant version of hemoglobin, contains fat-soluble vitamins, minerals, amino acids, and other valuable nutrients, and it appears to have antioxidant activity. It's available as a liquid extract (such as wheat grass extract), and it's present in spirulina and other edible blue-green algae.

Coenzyme Q10 (CoQ10) is not a free radical scavenger, but it helps prevent the formation of oxygen free radicals during cellular metabolism. Coenzyme Q10 is unique — and powerful — because it stops the inflammatory oxidation process before it begins by helping cells use oxygen more efficiently and produce fewer free radicals. This enzyme is present in every cell in the body, but its levels decrease with age. Supplementing with CoQ10 has been shown to improve oxygenation to the heart and may be beneficial in chronic inflammatory conditions such as cystitis and arthritis. Older pets, and those with inflammatory disease, may benefit from supplementation. A small dog should get 5 to 10 milligrams a day; large dogs up to 60 milligrams per day. The most bioavailable forms of CoQ10 are ubiquinone, ubiquinol, and Q-Gel.

Vitamin D has been the target of much research and media attention in the past decade. It turns out that this antioxidant vitamin is not so much a vitamin as a hormone, and it has wide-ranging effects on the body. Lack of vitamin D has been associated with everything from attention deficit/hyperactivity disorder to diabetes to cancer. Clearly, it's a very important nutrient — and its form is also important. Vitamin D3 (cholecalciferol) is the natural form; vitamin D_2 (ergocalciferol) is synthetic and should be avoided. Because dogs lack the mechanism in their skin that humans have to produce vitamin D, they must obtain it in their diet. Commercial pet foods are already plentifully supplemented with vitamin D; giving more may be harmful. Because it can easily reach toxic levels with supplementation, please consult with a veterinarian who is well versed in canine clinical nutrition before giving your dog additional vitamin D.

Açai is a tropical fruit loaded with flavonoid antioxidants that may have significant antiaging benefits. It contains amino acids and trace minerals that improve muscle tone and slow down the destructive effects to the skin. It also contains oleic acid, a fatty acid that helps keep cell membranes flexible.

Beta-glucans are polysaccharides (complex sugars), usually derived from mushrooms or yeast, with significant immune-boosting power. They are used to stimulate the immune system. While this supplement should not be used continuously, it can safely be used for several months when the immune system needs special support, such as while recovering from injury, surgery, or cancer therapy. Medicinal mushroom combinations (using species such as Reishi, Maitake, Tremella, Poria, and Polyporus) are concentrated sources of beta-glucans without the allergic potential of yeast.

Carotenoids are a large group of antioxidant plant pigments, including the following:

- *Astaxanthin:* These are red plant pigments with superior antioxidant capacity; dogs absorb them readily. They are used especially by infection-fighting white blood cells.
- *Beta-carotene:* Although dogs cannot convert beta-carotene to vitamin A, they can absorb it, and it may provide significant antioxidant benefits.
- *Lutein:* A yellow or orange pigment found in carrots, squash, and other orange and yellow fruits and vegetables as well as in green leafy vegetables such as spinach. Lutein is highly concentrated in the retinas and is important for good vision.
- *Lycopene:* Found most abundantly in tomatoes, lycopene is a fat-soluble red plant pigment with excellent antioxidant and cancer-fighting capabilities.

Flavonoids, a large group of antioxidants found in fruits and vegetables, have antiviral, antiallergic, antiplatelet, anti-inflammatory, and antitumor properties. Examples include the following:

- *Anthocyanadins and proanthocyanadins:* These red and blue plant pigments are found in blueberries, blackberries, raspberries, and strawberries.
- *Vitamin C:* Dogs make some vitamin C in their bodies, but given the forms of pollution (air, light, sound, electromagnetic) that we and our pets are exposed to daily, there are clear benefits of adding more to the diet. A vitamin C whole food complex is ideal because it contains many other helpful compounds.
- *Quercetin:* This well-studied antioxidant found in apples, grapefruit, grapes, blueberries, and broccoli has unique anticancer properties, and it blocks substances involved in allergies.

Silymarin and silybum are extracts of active ingredients of the milk thistle plant, which has been used for centuries to protect and heal the liver, the body's major detoxifying organ. A healthy liver is one of the best defenses against the aging effects of toxins.

Goji berries (*Lycium* spp.), also called wolfberries, are members of the nightshade family from the valleys of the Himalayas, renowned for its long-lived peoples. Goji berries contain a high concentration of anti-oxidants, including vitamin C, lutein, and selenium, as well as germanium sesquioxide, an organic mineral complex with significant anticancer properties. Known as the longevity fruit, goji berries are traditionally used to support kidney and liver function, fortify the bones, and enhance qi (chi), the basic life force.

MSM is a source of elemental sulfur, the third most abundant element in the body and a component of all connective tissues. Sulfur reserves decrease with age. MSM, besides having its own antioxidant activity, contributes to ongoing maintenance and repair in connective tissues including skin, cartilage, ligaments, and tendons. It is often combined with glucosamine for arthritis and joint pain.

OTHER SUPPLEMENTS

Protandim. We recommend a product for our Paleo Dogs called Protandim, which we also take ourselves. The company that makes the human version, LifeVantage, makes a chewable daily Protandim supplement for dogs called Canine Health. The formula starts with the same five botanical ingredients (listed below) as the human version, but also adds collagen, which has been studied for its positive effects on joint disease, and omega-3 fatty acids.

Milk thistle seed extract. Milk thistle has been used for centuries as a liver tonic. It has been extensively studied and shown to be safe and effective. Specifically, milk thistle protects the liver against toxins (including some molds such as aflatoxin, drugs, and heavy metals) and stimulates growth of new liver cells to replace those that are dead or damaged. Milk thistle has both powerful antioxidant and anti-inflammatory actions.

Bacopa extract (aerial part). Bacopa is generally used to enhance memory, learning, and concentration, and to help the body cope with stress. Research suggests that this adaptogenic herb may also have benefits for the respiratory, cardiovascular, and gastrointestinal systems. Bacopa is also considered to protect against free radical damage.

Ashwagandha (root). Sometimes called Indian ginseng, ashwaganda is widely used in Ayurvedic medicine. It has long been used as a tonic to improve overall health and reduce stress. It is an immune system booster with strong anti-inflammatory and antioxidant properties.

Green tea leaf extract. This common beverage herb from *Camellia sinensis* has many

442

beneficial effects. It is a good source of anti-oxidants, and research suggests it may help slow the growth of certain cancers.

Turmeric extract (rhizome). Besides being a popular culinary spice, turmeric is also a medicinal herb with powerful antioxidant properties. It has been studied for its benefits on inflammation related to joint discomfort, liver problems, viral infections, and cardiovascular and gastrointestinal conditions.

Garlic. While dogs love it, garlic is in the same family as onions, and in large doses it can be toxic, especially to little dogs. We do not recommend raw garlic or culinary garlic (granulated, salt, or powder). We recommend Kyolic brand garlic. But do not over-supplement with Kyolic. Use only one drop per pound of meat.

Choline, also known as phosphatidylcholine, is a member of the B vitamin group that is helpful for older dogs who seem to be losing their memory or becoming a bit senile. It improves brain function and cognition.

Colostrum, also called first milk, is the thin yellowish fluid produced by mammary glands prior to real milk and makes up the first few meals for the newborn. Colostrum is full of antibodies, growth factors, enzymes, immune factors, hormones, and micronutrients; it provides the young with immunity while their own immune systems are still developing. Cows produce large amounts of colostrum, and this is the source for most commercial formulations. It has been used to treat allergies, cancer, colitis, diarrhea, poor wound healing, and many types of infection. Colostrum could be called the first antiaging supplement, since it is the first food of all mammal babies.

Willard Water (Dr. Willard's Water, catalyzed altered water) acts as a normalizer on all living things not in a healthy state. Willard Water can help assimilate nutrients more efficiently, increase enzyme activity, and strengthen the immune system. Always dilute it according to the directions.

Super blue-green algae are a wonderful source of concentrated nutrition. Note that not all algae are safe to consume; there are many types of toxic algae as well as health-giving species such as kelp, dulse, and nori. Algae grown in lakes under natural conditions may become contaminated with bacteria and heavy metals. Nutritive blue-green algae include spirulina, chlorella, and many others.

The products we recommend are BioSuperfood, which can be used for humans and animals, and the specific pet formulation BioPreparation. Both contain four species of microalgae (*Spirulina pacifica, Spirulina platensis, Dunaliella salina,* and *Haematococcus pluvialis*) that offer a full spectrum of highly bioavailable, concentrated nutrients: vitamins, minerals, amino acids, essential fatty acids, natural antioxidants (including astaxanthin, chlorophyll, and phycocyanin), and more than 400 enzymes. While the potency of the nutrients is low, compared with most vitamin supplements, their maximal bioavailability make them powerful high-dose supplements. BioSuperfood and BioPreparation are different from other popular algae products like spirulina and chlorella because the four species in these products have polysaccharide cell walls, while most other algae have indigestible cellulose cell walls. This makes BioSuperfood and BioPreparation much easier to digest and absorb, which is particularly valuable for those with digestive problems. BioPreparation is highly palatable, and even fussy dogs will eat the powder without complaint when it's mixed with their wet food (canned or homemade); the capsules are quite small and easy to administer whole. However, it's wise to start with just a tiny bit, because it's extremely powerful, and too much may detoxify your pet more quickly than is comfortable for either of you.

BioSuperfood and BioPreparation algae are grown hydroponically under strictly controlled laboratory standards using water that comes directly from an underground volcanic spring. Independent laboratory testing assures the products' freedom from all chemicals, pesticides, herbicides, heavy metals, bacteria, and other contaminants (including radiation).

Here are just some of the benefits that have been seen with BioSuperfood and Bio-Preparation in animals and humans.

- Improved digestion and assimilation of nutrients
- Increased appetite and interest in eating new foods
- Weight loss
- Supple, healthy skin or glossy fur
- Relief of arthritis pain, asthma, inflammatory bowel disease (IBD), and other inflammatory conditions
- Increased mobility in older animals
- Increased stamina and overall energy
- Sounder sleep
- Quicker healing
- Shorter recovery time after surgery
- Fewer and briefer colds and infections

- More balanced emotions (leading to improved behavior)
- Balanced growth and development
- Enhanced blood cell development
- Cancers and tumors prevented and reduced

What may be most interesting about Bio-Superfood and BioPreparation is their ability to create synergism with food and even medications. Digestion and absorption are greatly enhanced, meaning that your pet will get more nutrition from food. The amount of medications your pet may be taking, including herbs, can often be reduced. (Be sure to work with your veterinarian to adjust the dosage as your pet's system gets healthier.)

APPENDIX B:
FOOD-BORNE DISEASES

As discussed in Chapter 9, much is made of the issue of bacterial contamination in the meat likely to be used in homemade raw diets — i.e., meat from the grocery store. And the naysayers have a point: There's no doubt that the U.S. meat supply is pretty dirty. Meat safety falls under the Hazard Analysis and Critical Control Points (HACCP) system; unfortunately, it more or less leaves cleanliness up to the people who run the slaughterhouses. You can imagine how successful that method has been! A new system of irradiation is being introduced to kill the gazillions of pathogenic bacteria on all of those feces-smeared carcasses — because *preventing* feces from being smeared all over them in the first place would be too much trouble.

It should be noted that in most of the studies of raw meat diets done to date, the authors were highly motivated to discredit and disparage raw diets. That they haven't been terribly successful speaks volumes about the practical risk, which drops to nearly nothing when the procedures outlined in Chapter 8 (including standard safe meat handling and sanitizing raw meat and bones) are followed.

Let's look specifically at all the nasty things in raw meat that veterinarians worry about. An article published by Dr. Narda Robinson of Colorado State University offers a litany of scary bugs that can kill not only your dog but maybe you and your whole family, too.[1] We'll start with the most common ones and go from there.

Salmonella **spp.** These notorious bacteria are a very common contaminant of raw meat, raw poultry, and raw eggs. They have been well studied by many researchers. According to one study, "*Salmonella* was isolated from 80 percent of the BARF [bones and raw food or biologically appropriate raw food] diet samples ($P < 0.001$) and from 30 percent of the stool samples from dogs fed the diet ($P = 0.105$). Dogs fed raw chicken may therefore be a source of environmental contamination."[2] However, this study looked at only 20 dogs (10 raw-fed, 10 on a control diet), and of the three positive stool samples, only one was from a dog whose food contained the same serovar; another was from a dog whose food contained a different serovar; and the last was from a dog whose food tested negative. No dog or human illness was reported, despite confirmed contamination of the food. This has consistently been the case with nearly every analysis of raw foods: They contain plenty of pathogens, but nobody is getting sick.

The literature supports the fact that zoonotic transmission of *Salmonella* from pets to people is extremely rare. A 2011 review found only a single U.S. case of transmission of *Salmonella* from a dog to a human since 1974 — and in that case, the human let the dog eat broth that had been standing, unrefrigerated, for days.[3]

Another study states that 95 percent of human *Salmonella* cases are due to people eating contaminated food. The authors speculate that some number of these could be due to contact with dogs or dog food, and cite data from 1987 estimating that 1 percent of human salmonellosis *could* be due to contact with pets (but not pet food). The authors conclude, "To date, raw pet foods have not been associated with salmonellosis in humans."[4]

The same cannot be said for commercial pet food. There have been dozens of recalls of dry dog food due to *Salmonella* contamination. In one 2012 outbreak, more than four dozen people became ill from merely handling dry dog food. That's pretty hefty contamination, if you ask us.

Research suggests that up to 36 percent of dogs and 18 percent of cats are asymptomatic carriers of *Salmonella*.[5] The possible source of the organism isn't discussed, but would include the environment as well as diet — which is, of course, most likely to be heat-processed pet food, since that's what is eaten by 90 percent of U.S. dogs.[6]

Dogs themselves appear to be quite resistant to illness due to this ubiquitous bacteria.[7] The evidence clearly shows that *Salmonella,* the most common pathogen of raw-meat diets, is not a significant threat to human or animal health.

Campylobacter. This bacteria is also a very common contaminant of U.S. meat and poultry. However, no alarm was raised about it until someone developed a test for it — then, lo and behold, it was everywhere!

There has been one study of the public health risks of feeding a raw diet to dogs.[8] As evidence, this review cites a Hungarian study that included free-roaming dogs that had access to aborted livestock fetuses and raw poultry that were found to be contaminated with *Campylobacter*. One person became sick, but it is unknown whether he himself handled the infected tissues.

Further research suggests that only a "small proportion of human infections are acquired from dogs . . . usually [from] puppies that are themselves suffering from diarrhoea. Only four infections associated with cats (all kittens with diarrhoea) have been reported." The study concludes that dogs and cats are unlikely to be the source of human infections.[9] Phylogenetic analysis of cases, which are strongly seasonal, suggests that most human cases of campylobacteriosis are most likely due to water contamination.[10]

Another study on *Campylobacter* states that "if a person and a pet have concurrent campylobacteriosis, the veterinarian must consider whether they both obtained it from some other common source (for example, food or water) or if the pet obtained it from the human being." The authors conclude that dogs and cats are unlikely to be the source of human infection.[11]

Toxoplasma gondii. This protozoal parasite may encyst in raw meat. Cats are the definitive host for this organism, meaning that it can only grow and reproduce in cats. Other species can become infected, but they do not shed infectious cysts. Adult dogs are rarely infected, although puppies are more susceptible. The primary cause of human toxoplasmosis is humans themselves consuming raw or undercooked meat, milk, or shellfish.[12]

In Canada and some other countries, *Toxoplasma* is a common contaminant of pork.[13] However, raw diet proponents (ourselves included) do not recommend feeding uncooked pork, and no raw diet studied to date has contained pork.

Clostridium perfringens. These bacteria, commonly found in decaying vegetation, are common and contagious causes of gastroenteritis in dogs and cats. Infections are usually self-limiting. One study states, "No associations between *C. difficile, MRSA,* or *VRE* and consumption of raw meat were detected." So, not only is *C. perfringens* not a serious issue, but also neither is the more virulent *C. difficile.*

Clostridium botulinum. Long before Botox became a miracle anti-aging drug, the toxins produced by this organism were better known for causing a degenerative paralytic and usually fatal disease called botulism. It has been documented in hunting dogs,[14] and in another case, two dogs from the same owner were referred for suspected botulism. Those dogs had been fed expired canned food (canned goods are a common source of botulism); they were also allowed to roam and may have eaten a contaminated carcass.[15]

Neospora caninum. This very common pathogen of cattle was, until 1988, misidentified as *Toxoplasma.* It can cause serious disease in young or immunocompromised dogs. As with *Toxoplasma,* freezing kills the cysts.[16]

E. coli. The U.S. meat supply, particularly beef, is highly contaminated with *E. coli.* The organism is also ubiquitous in the environment. People commonly carry it. In the vast majority of cases, *E. coli* is a harmless commensal (part of the normal bacterial population) of the gastro-intestinal tract. A study that looked for a pathogenic strain, *E. coli* O157, in dogs fed raw meat and in their environment found none.[17]

Listeria monocytogenes. This is a very common cause of food poisoning in humans. Virtually all human listeria is due to consumption of contaminated foods such as meat, cheese, or milk. However, contamination occurs during the processing of these foods for cold cuts, hot dogs, and similar products. The literature reports listeriosis in one dog, source unknown. There is no evidence that any human or pet has ever contracted *Listeria* from fresh, raw meats.

Staphylococcus aureus. These enterprising, toxin-producing organisms can be found in raw meat as well as commercially prepared foods, among many other places. They may proliferate and produce toxins if the food is allowed to sit out. This is why we recommend that meals be left out for only a short period of time.

Many digestive upsets of dogs may be related to bacterial growth in moist food put out for dogs and left for many hours before being eaten. Moreover, many people mix water, broth, or other liquids with dry dog foods; this is clearly risky, given the level of bacteria known to inhabit the surface of dry food.

In the United States, *Staph* contamination of meat is thought to come from food animals themselves and not their processing. It's documented to occur in pigs in the United States and elsewhere, and to infect workers.[18]

The possibility of transmission of *S. aureus* between humans and dogs has been investigated. The organism was found in the nasal cavities of 24 percent of the people but less than 9 percent of the dogs, and there was a strong association between the person being in a health-care-related occupation and the presence of S. aureus.[19] This bacteria is also a common cause of skin infections in dogs. However, there are no reported cases of dogs contracting S. aureus from raw meat.

Bacillus cereus. One researcher conducted tests on more than 40 brands of dry dog food. Every food sample tested positive for B. cereus. The study's author attributes most cases of "garbage gut" to B. cereus, not to Staph.[20]

Yersinia enterocolitica. This mild-mannered relative of Yersinia pestis (the infamous cause of bubonic plague) is considered a normal commensal in dogs and is widespread in the environment.[21] Raw meat is not likely to be a significant source of infection.

Most of the other organisms referenced by Dr. Robinson are more theoretical risks than practical ones. A dog could get many diseases from eating dead wild animals like rabbits, bears, and walruses; 4-D (dead, dying, diseased, or disabled) slaughterhouse waste; or raw horsemeat, raw fish, or raw pork — all of which we strongly recommend against! Moreover, the meat-sanitizing procedures outlined in Chapter 8 are an additional safeguard against such diseases. Nevertheless, we want to be thorough and address all possible infectious organisms.

Francisella tularensis. An endemic disease in wild rabbits, beavers, and muskrats.

Mycobacterium bovis **and** *M. tuberculinum.* These may be present in the organ meat of infected animals.

Burkholderia (Pseudomonas) pseudomallei. Causes glanders disease of horses.

Rabies. Yes, rabid animals die, and yes, a dog could eat the carcass, cut its mouth on a bone, and get infected with rabies through the wound. This is very unlikely.

Pseudorabies (Aujeszky's disease). A disease of swine documented to have occurred in seven dogs in Spain who ate diseased pig lungs.

Trichinella spiralis. A parasite of pork, walrus, seal, and bear meat, none of which we recommend.

Diphyllobothrium latum, Opisthorchis tenuicollis, Dioctophyme renale, **and** *Nanophyetus salmincola* **(the vector of** *Neorickettsia helminthoeca).* These are all parasites of raw fish, which we do not recommend.

Sarcocystis **spp.** *Sarcocystis* is not considered to be of pathologic significance in most animals.

***Taenia* and *Echinococcus* spp.** Tapeworms that, if present in livestock at slaughter, will result in the carcass being condemned for human consumption (although diseased organs and carcasses are allowed by the FDA to be processed into dry dog food).

Toxocara canis. The common dog roundworm, most commonly contracted from mothers' milk or dirt.

Baylisascaris procyonis. A roundworm that infects raccoons and is considered to be a significant human health hazard, particularly for children who may contract it through contact with a raccoon "latrine."

Perhaps the risk associated with zoonotic disease was summarized best by Kahrs et al.: "The transmission of pet-borne zoonoses is complex and usually requires close contact between susceptible human beings and animals or their excretions. Such contact frequently involves lack of common sense and gross breach of sound hygienic practice."[22] We believe our readers have good sense and will understand the importance of sound hygiene and meat handling procedures.

On the flip side, there are multiple studies

showing that raw meat diets for pets are more digestible than heat-processed foods.[23]

A board-certified veterinary nutritionist who was previously a researcher at a major pet food company stated that she had studied raw diets and that animals did better on raw diets than processed ones.[24] We suspect that all the big pet food companies have done similar research and have their own raw diet formulations waiting to be marketed when they are assured of making a profit on them.

ENDNOTES

Chapter 1

1 "Tooth Found in Cave of Orce Named Earliest Human Remain," *Olive Press,* March 9, 2013, http://www.theolivepress .es/spain-news/2013/03/09/tooth-found-in-cave-of-orce-named-earliest-human-remain.

2 DP Laflamme, SK Abood, AJ Fascetti, et al., "Pet Feeding Practices of Dog and Cat Owners in the United States and Australia," *Journal of the American Veterinary Medical Association* 232, no. 5 (2008): 687–94.

3 CA Kirk, "Preventing Obesity in Dogs and Cats," *World Small Animal Veterinary Association World Congress Proceedings* 2011.

4 "Periodontal Disease," American Veterinary Dental College, http://www.avdc.org/ periodontaldisease.html.

5 National Canine Cancer Foundation, http://www.wearethecure.org/more_cancer_facts.htm.

6 LD Mech, *Wolves: Behavior, Ecology, and Conservation* (Chicago: University of Chicago Press, 2007).

7 C Chambreau, *The Healthy Animal's Journal,* http://www.christinachambreau.com.

8 M Davies, "Geriatric Screening in First Opinion Practice — Results from 45 Dogs," *Journal of Small Animal Practice* 53, no. 9 (September 2012): 507–13, doi:10.1111/j.1748-5827.2012.01247.

9 "Fat Pets Are Getting Fatter, According to Latest Survey," Association for Pet Obesity Prevention, February 23, 2011, http://www.petobesity prevention.com/fat-pets-getting-fatter-according-to-latest-survey.

10 MS Hand, CD Thatcher, RL Remillard, et al., *Small Animal Clinical Nutrition,* 4th ed. (Topeka, Kansas: Mark Morris Association 2000).

11 "Nestlé Purina Study Confirms Link between Body Fat, Certain Health Conditions," *DVM 360 Magazine,* January 1, 2004.

12 *Super Size Me,* directed by Morgan Spurlock (2004; Kathbur Pictures).

13 U.S. Food and Drug Administration,

Compliance Policy Guide Sec. 675.400 Rendered Animal Feed Ingredients, http://www.fda.gov/ICECI/ComplianceManuals/CompliancePolicyGuidanceManual/ucm074717.htm; and Association of American Feed Control Officials, *Official Publication,* 2013.

14 M Lenoir, F Serre, L Cantin, et al., "Intense Sweetness Surpasses Cocaine Reward," *PLoS ONE* 2, no. 8,doi:10.1371/journal.pone.0000698.

15 RI Issa and TM Griffin, "Pathobiology of Obesity and Osteoarthritis: Integrating Biomechanics and Inflammation," *Pathobiology of Aging and Age Related Diseases* 2 (May 9, 2012): 17470, http://www.ncbi.nlm.nih.gov/pmc/articles/PMC3364606.

16 RCM Van Kruijsdijk, E van der Wall, and FLJ Visseren, "Obesity and Cancer: The Role of Dysfunctional Adipose Tissue," *Cancer Epidemiology Biomarkers Prevention* 18 (2009): 2569–78, http://cebp.aacrjournals.org/content/18/10/2569.full.pdf.

17 EC Westman, RD Feinman, JC Mavropoulos, et al., "Low-Carbohydrate Nutrition and Metabolism," *American Journal of Clinical Nutrition* 86 (2007): 276–84, http://ajcn.nutrition.org/content/86/2/276.full.pdf.

18 DE Linder and LM Freeman, "Evaluation of Calorie Density and Feeding Directions for Commercially Available Diets Designed for Weight Loss in Dogs and Cats," *Journal of the American Veterinary Medical Association* 236, no. 1 (January 1, 2010): 74–77.

19 P Nguyen, H Domon, V Biourge, et al., "Glycemic and Insulinemic Responses after Ingestion of Commercial Foods in Healthy Dogs: Influence of Food Composition," *Journal of Nutrition* 128, no. 12 (December 1, 1998): 2654S–58S.

20 M Diez, P Nguyen, I Jeusette, et al., "Weight Loss in Obese Dogs: Evaluation of a High-Protein, Low-Carbohydrate Diet," *Journal of Nutrition* 132, no. 6 (June 1, 2002): 1685S–87S.

21 JA Ello-Martin, LS Roe, JH Ledikwe, et al., "Dietary Energy Density in the Treatment of Obesity: A Year-Long Trial Comparing 2 Weight-Loss Diets," *American Journal of Clinical Nutrition* 85, no. 6 (June 2007): 1465–77.

22 HK Sivertsen, O Ueland, and F Westad, "Development of Satiating and Palatable High-Protein Meat Products by Using Experimental Design in Food Technology," *Food and Nutrition Research* 54 (2010): 5114.

23 WD Cusick, *Canine Nutrition (Revised): Choosing the Best Food for Your Breed of Dog* (Irvine, California: Doral Publishing, 1997), http://www.wdcusick.com/2.pdf.

24 E Axelsson, A Ratnakumar, ML Arendt, et al., "The Genomic Signature of Dog Domestication Reveals Adaptation to a Starch-Rich Diet," *Nature* 490 (March 21, 2013): 360–64, doi:10.1038/nature11837.

Chapter 2

1 K Lindblad-Toh, CM Wade, TS Mikkelsen, et al., "Genome Sequence, Comparative Analysis and Haplotype Structure of the Domestic Dog," *Nature* 438 (December 8, 2005): 803–19.

2 AS Druzhkova, O Thalmann, VA Trifonov, et al., "Ancient DNA Analysis Affirms the Canid from Altai as a Primitive Dog," *PLoS ONE* 8, no. 3 (2013): e57754, doi:10.1371/journal.pone.0057754.

3 K Lord, "A Comparison of the Sensory Development of Wolves (*Canis lupus lupus*) and Dogs (*Canis lupus familiaris*)," *Ethology* 119, no. 2 (February 2013): 110–20.

4 L Trut, "Early Canid Domestication: The Farm-Fox Experiment," *American Scientist* 87 (March–April 1999): 160–69.

5 ZL Ding, M Oskarsson, A Ardalan, et al., "Origins of Domestic Dog in Southern East Asia Is Supported by Analysis of Y-Chromosome DNA," *Heredity* 108, no. 5 (May 2012): 507–14.

6 M Poptsova, S Banerjee, O Gokcumen, et al., "Impact of Constitutional Copy Number Variants on Biological Pathway Evolution," *BioMed Central Evolutionary Biology* 13 (2013): 19–31.

7 GH Perry, NJ Dominy, KG Claw, et al., "Diet and the Evolution of Human Amylase Gene Copy Number Variation," *Nature Genetics* 39, no. 10 (October 2007): 1256–60.

8 E Axelsson, A Ratnakumar, ML Arendt, et al., "The Genomic Signature of Dog Domestication Reveals Adaptation to a Starch-Rich Diet," *Nature* (2013, in press), doi:10.1038/nature11837.

9 EO Price, *Animal Domestication and Behavior* (New York: CABI Publishing, 2002).

10 JP Scott, *Dog Behavior: The Genetic Basis* (Chicago: University of Chicago Press, 1974), 55–56.

11 American Kennel Club, http://www.akc.org/breeds/index.cfm.

1 LJ DeBowes, D Mosier, E Logan et al., "Association of Periodontal Disease and Histologic Lesions in Multiple Organs from 45 Dogs." *Journal of Veterinary Dentistry* 13, no. 2 (June 1996): 57–60.

2 F Colyer, "Dental Disease in Animals," *British Dental Journal* 82 (1947): 31–35.

3 MG Brown and JF Park, "Control of Dental Calculus in Experimental Beagles," *Laboratory Animal Care* 18, no. 5 (October 1968): 527–35.

4 CJ Lopez-Bote, R Sanz Arias, AI Rey, et al., "Effect of Free-Range Feeding on Omega-3 Fatty Acids and Alpha-Tocopherol Content and Oxidative Stability of Eggs," *Animal Feed Science and Technology* 72 (1998): 33–40.

5 C Ip, JA Scimeca, and HJ Thompason, "Conjugated Linoleic Acid: A Powerful Anti-Carcinogen from Animal Fat Sources," *Cancer* 1, suppl. 3 (August 1, 1994): 1050–54.

6 P French, C Stanton, F Lawless, et al., "Fatty Acid Composition, Including Conjugated Linoleic Acid, of Intramuscular Fat from Steers Offered Grazed Grass, Grass Silage, or Concentrate-Based Diets," *Journal of Animal Science* 78, no. 11

(November 2000): 2849–55.

7 R Heuberger, "Save Money with Home-made Dog Food," *Bark,* http://www.the bark.com/content/save-money-home made-dog-food.

8 KK Barnowe-Meyer, PJ White, TL Davis, et al., "Influences of Wolves and High-Elevation Dispersion on Reproductive Success of Pronghorn (*Antilocapra americana*)," *Journal of Mammalogy* 91, no. 3 (2010): 712–21.

9 RL Beschtal and WJ Ripple, "Recovering Riparian Plant Communities with Wolves in Northern Yellowstone," *Restoration Ecology* 18, no. 3 (May 2010): 380–89.

10 FM Pottenger, *Pottenger's Cats: A Study in Nutrition,* 2nd ed. (San Diego: Price-Pottenger Foundation, 1995).

11 MW Fox, *Eating with Conscience: The Bioethics of Food* (Troutdale, Oregon: NewSage Press, 1997).

Chapter 4

1 U.S. Food and Drug Administration, Compliance Policy Guide, http://www.fda .gov/ICECI/ComplianceManuals/Com pliancePolicyGuidanceManual/ucm0747 17.htm.

2 Ibid.

3 Association of American Feed Control Officials, *Official Publication,* 2013 (West Lafayette, Indiana: AAFCO, 2013).

4 JG Morris and QR Rogers, "Assessment of the Nutritional Adequacy of Pet Foods Through the Life Cycle," *Journal of Nutrition* 124 (1994): 2520S–34S.

5 RA Burns, MH LeFaivre, and JA Milner, "Effects of Dietary Protein Quantity and Quality on the Growth of Dogs and Rats," *Journal of Nutrition* 112 (1982): 1845–53.

6 LP Case and GL Czarnecki-Maulden, "Protein Requirements of Growing Pups Fed Practical Dry-Type Diets Containing Mixed-Protein Sources," *American Journal of Veterinary Research* 51, no. 5 (May 1990): 808–12.

7 Ibid.

8 FDA, "Compliance Policy Guides: Sec. 675.400 Rendered Animal Feed Ingredients," http://www.fda.gov/ICECI/ComplianceManuals/CompliancePolicyGuidanceManual/ucm074717.htm.

9 Dog Cancer Vet, http://dogcancervet.com.

10 IM Berquin, IJ Edwards, and YQ Chen, "Multi-Targeted Therapy of Cancer by Omega-3 Fatty Acids," *Cancer Letters* 269, no. 2 (October 8, 2008): 363–77, doi: 10.1016/j.canlet.2008.03.044.

11 DM Vail, GK Ogilvie, SL Wheeler, et al., "Alterations in Carbohydrate Metabolism in Canine Lymphoma," *Journal of Veterinary Internal Medicine* 4, no. 1 (January–February 1990): 8–11.

12 VW Ho, K Leung, A Hsu, et al., "A Low Carbohydrate, High Protein Diet Slows Tumor Growth and Prevents Cancer Initiation," *Cancer Research* 71, no. 13 (July 1, 2011): 4484–93, doi: 10.1158/0008-5472.CAN-10-3973.

13 EC Westman, RD Feinman, JC Mavropoulos, et al., "Low-Carbohydrate Nutrition and Metabolism," *American Journal of Clinical Nutrition* 86 (2007): 276–84, http://ajcn.nutrition.org/content/86/2/276.full.pdf.

14 Association of American Feed Control Officials, *Official Publication,* 2013, 452–60.

15 Environmental Working Group, "Polluted Pets: High Levels of Toxic Industrial Chemicals Contaminate Dogs and Cats," April 17, 2008, http://www.ewg.org/research/polluted-pets.

16 Pew Campaign on Human Health and Industrial Farming, "Record-High Antibiotic Sale for Livestock Production," February 6, 2013, http://www.pewhealth.org/reports-analysis/data-visualizations/record-

high-antibiotic-sales-for-meat-and-poultry-production-85899449165.

17 FDA and the Center for Veterinary Medicine, "Report on the Risk from Pentobarbital in Dog Food," March 1, 2001, http://www.fda.gov/AboutFDA/CentersOffices/OfficeofFoods/CVM/CVMFOIAElectronicReadingRoom/ucm129131.htm.

18 JS de Vendômois, F Roullier, D Cellier, and G-E Séralini,. "A Comparison of the Effects of Three GM Corn Varieties on Mammalian Health," *International Journal of Biological Sciences* 5, no. 7 (2009): 706–26, doi:10.7150/ijbs.5.706, http://www.ijbs.com/v05p0706.htm.

19 M Antoniou, C Robinson, and J Fagan, "GMO Myths and Truths: An Evidence-Based Examination of the Claims Made for the Safety and Efficacy of Genetically Modified Crops," Earth Open Source, June 2012, http://earthopensource.org/files/pdfs/GMO_Myths_and_Truths/GMO_Myths_and_Truths_1.3b.pdf.

20 E Lau, "Cats Susceptible to Neurological Problems When Fed Irradiated Diets," Veterinary Information Network News Service, June 8, 2009.

21 SS Epstein and W Hauter, "Preventing Pathogenic Food Poisoning: Sanitation,

Not Irradiation," *International Journal of Health Services* 31, no. 1 (2001): 187–92.

22 "More Aflatoxin-Related Dog Food Recalls Revealed," *Food Safety News,* December 29, 2011, http://www.food safetynews.com/2011/12/more-aflatoxin-related-dog-food-recalls-revealed/#.UV XuYFtAR40.

23 Association of American Feed Control Officials, *Official Publication,* 2013, 424.

24 "US Petfood Import and Export Trends," PetFood Industry.com, April 27, 2011, http://www.petfoodindustry.com/ Default.aspx?pageid=5306&id=7100& terms=china+imports.

Chapter 5

1 SD Meola, CC Tearney, SA Haas et al., "Evaluation of Trends in Marijuana Toxicosis in Dogs Living in a State with Legalized Medical Marijuana: 125 Dogs (2005–2010)." *Journal of Veterinary Emergency and Critical Care* 22, no. 6 (December 2012): 690–96.

2 Environmental Working Group, "Polluted Pets: High Levels of Toxic Industrial Chemicals Contaminate Cats and Dogs," April 17, 2008, http://www.ewg.org/book/

export/html/26238, accessed January 11, 2013.

3 KM Ng, JA Ferrevra, SK Higginbottom, et al., "Microbiota-Liberated Host Sugars Facilitate Post-Antibiotic Expansion of Enteric Pathogens," *Nature* (2013), online publication in advance of print, http://dx .doi.org/10.1038/nature12503.

4 International Veterinary Academy of Pain Management, http://www.ivapm.org.

5 A Wagner and P Hellyer, "Survey of Anesthesia Techniques and Concerns in Private Veterinary Practice," *Journal of the American Veterinary Medical Association* 217, no. 11 (December 1, 2000): 1652–57.

6 LJ Sanborn, "Long-Term Health Risks and Benefits Associated with Spay/Neuter in Dogs," National Animal Interest Alliance, 2007, http://www.naiaonline.org/ pdfs/LongTermHealthEffectsOfSpayNeu terInDogs.pdf.

7 HJ McSorley, JP Hewitson, and RM Maizels, "Immunomodulation by Helminth Parasites: Defining Mechanisms and Mediators," *International Journal for Parasitology* 43 (January 3, 2013): 301–10.

8 TK Fuller, "Population Dynamics of Wolves in North-Central Minnesota," *Wildlife Society Wildlife Monographs* no.

105 (1989): 41.

9 DH Knight and JB Lok, "Seasonality of Heartworm Infection and Implications for Chemoprophylaxis," *Clinical Techniques in Small Animal Practice* 13, no. 2 (May 1998): 77–82.

10 DD Bowman, "Heartworms, Macrocyclic Lactones, and the Specter of Resistance to Prevention in the United States," *Parasites and Vectors* 5 (July 9, 2012): 138.

11 L Hardell, M Carlberg, and K Hansson Mild, "Use of Mobile Phones and Cordless Phones Is Associated with Increased Risk for Glioma and Acoustic Neuroma," *Pathophysiology* 20, no. 2 (December 20, 2012): 85–110.

12 L Hardell and C Sage, "Biological Effects from Electromagnetic Field Exposure and Public Exposure Standards," *Biomedicine and Pharmacotherapy* 62, no. 2 (February 2008): 104–9.

13 GW Hacker, E Pawlak, G Pauser, et al., "Biomedical Evidence of Influence of Geopathic Zones on the Human Body: Scientifically Traceable Effects and Ways of Harmonization," *Forschende Komplementärmedizin und Klassische Naturheilkunde (Research in Complementary and*

Natural Classical Medicine) 12, no. 6 (December 2005): 315–27.

Chapter 6

1 ES Almberg, PC Cross, AP Dobson, et al., "Parasite Invasion Following Host Reintroduction: A Case Study of Yellowstone's Wolves," *Philosophical Transactions of the Royal Society B* 367, no. 164 (2012): 2840–51.

2 TR Phillips and RD Schultz, "Canine and Feline Vaccines," in *Current Veterinary Therapy* 11, ed. by RW Kirk and JD Bonagura (Philadelphia: W.B. Saunders Co., 1992), 202–6.

3 LV Wellborn, JG DeVries, R Ford, et al., "AAHA Canine Vaccination Guidelines," *Journal of the American Animal Hospital Association* 47, no. 5 (September–October 2011): 1–42.

4 H HogenEsch, J Azcona-Olivera, C Scott-Moncrieff, et al., "Vaccine-Induced Autoimmunity in the Dog," *Advances in Veterinary Medicine* 47 (1999): 733–47.

5 JC Scott-Moncrieff, J Azcona-Olivera, NW Glickman, et al., "Evaluation of Antithyroglobulin Antibodies after Routine Vaccination in Pet and Research Dogs," *Journal of the American Veterinary Medical*

Association 221, no. 4 (August 15, 2002): 515–21.

6 JS Rand, LM Fleeman, HA Farrow, et al., "Canine and Feline Diabetes Mellitus: Nature or Nurture?" University of Queensland, Center for Companion Animal Health, http://www.uq.edu.au/ccah/index.html?page=43608&pid=0.

7 K Tsumiyama, Y Miyazaki, and S Shiozawa, "Self-Organized Criticality Theory of Autoimmunity," *PLoS ONE* 4, no. 12 (2009): e8382, doi:10.1371/journal.pone.0008382.

8 RH Pitcairn, "A New Look at the Vaccine Question," *Proceedings of the Annual Conference of the American Holistic Veterinary Medical Association,* 1993.

9 JM Modlin, "The Bumpy Road to Polio Eradication," *New England Journal of Medicine* 362 (2010): 2346–49.

10 A Dearment, "PhRMA Report Lists Almost 300 Vaccines under Development," *Drug Store News,* April 26, 2012, http://drug storenews.com/article/phrma-report-lists-almost-300-vaccines-under-development.

11 D Ramey, "Animal Vaccinations," Science-Based Medicine, 2009, http://www.sciencebasedmedicine.org/index.php/animal-vaccinations.

12 H HogenEsch, S Thompson, A Dunham, et al., "Effect of Age on Immune Parameters and the Immune Response of Dogs to Vaccines — Sectional Study," *Veterinary Immunology and Immunopathology* 97, nos. 1–2 (January 2004): 77–85.

13 GE Moore, LF Guptill, MP Ward, et al., "Adverse Events Diagnosed within Three Days of Vaccine Administration in Dogs," *Journal of the American Veterinary Medical Association* 227, no. 7 (October 1, 2005): 1102–8.

14 RD Schultz, B Thiel, E Mukhtar, et al., "Age and Long-Term Protective Immunity in Dogs and Cats," *Journal of Comparative Pathology* 142, suppl. 1 (January 2010): S102–8.

15 R Blaylock, "What to Do If Force Vaccinated," August 19, 2009, http://vactruth.com/2009/08/19/russell-blaylock-md-what-to-do-if-force-vaccinated.

Chapter 7

1 E Boden and GP West, *Black's Veterinary Dictionary* (Lanham, Maryland: Rowman and Littlefield, 1998).

2 National Research Council, *Nutrient Requirements of Dogs and Cats* (Washington, DC: National Academies Press,

2006); and LI Chiba, *Animal Nutrition Handbook* (Auburn, Alabama: Auburn University, 1999), 42.

3 AW Kotula, JP Dubey, AK Sharar, et al., "Effect of Freezing on Infectivity of *Toxoplasma gondii* Tissue Cysts in Pork," *Journal of Food Protection* 54 (September 1991): 687–90.

4 RK Buddington, "Postnatal Changes in Bacterial Populations in the Gastrointestinal Tract of Dogs," *American Journal of Veterinary Research* 64, no. 5 (May 2003): 646–51.

5 FDA and the Center for Veterinary Medicine, "Report on the Risk from Pentobarbital in Dog Food," March 1, 2001.

6 EA Ross, NJ Szabo, and IR Tebbett, "Lead Content of Calcium Supplements," *Journal of the American Medical Association* 284, no. 11 (2000): 1425–29.

Chapter 8

1 *"Canis lupus"* and *"Canis latrans,"* Animal Diversity Web, University of Michigan Museum of Zoology, http://animaldiversity .ummz.umich.edu/accounts/Canis_lupus; and "Red Fox," Wildlife Online, http:// www.wildlifeonline.me.uk/red_fox.html #longevity.

2 K Dammrich, "Relationship between Nutrition and Bone Growth in Large and Giant Dogs," *Journal of Nutrition* 121 (1991): 114S–21S.

Chapter 9

1 E Axelsson, A Ratnakumar, ML Arendt, et al., "The Genomic Signature of Dog Domestication Reveals Adaptation to a Starch-Rich Diet," *Nature* 495 (March 2013): 360–64, doi:10.1038/nature11837.

2 L Trut, "Early Canid Domestication: The Farm-Fox Experiment," *American Scientist* 87 (March–April 1999): 160–69.

3 J Cairns, "The Origin of Mutants," *Nature* 335, no. 6186 (September 8, 1988): 142–45.

4 HD Anderson, CA Elvehjem, and JE Gonce Jr., "A Comparison of the Nutritive Values of Raw, Pasteurized and Evaporated Milks for the Dog," *Journal of Nutrition* 20 (1940): 433–43.

5 C Miglio, E Chavaro, A Visconte, et al., "Effects of Different Cooking Methods on Nutritional and Physicochemical Characteristics of Selected Vegetables," *Journal of Agricultural Food Chemistry* 56 (2008): 139–47.

6 U.S. Department of Agriculture, Agricul-

tural Research Service, USDA National Nutrient Database for Standard Reference, Release 25, 2012, http://ndb.nal.usda.gov.

7 AF Morgan and GE Kern, "The Effect of Heat upon the Biological Value of Meat Protein," *Journal of Nutrition* 7, no. 4 (April 1934): 367–79.

8 SM Murray, AR Patil, GC Fahey, et al., "Raw and Rendered Animal By-Products as Ingredients in Dog Diets," *Journal of Animal Science* 75 (1997): 2497–505.

9 AF Morgan and GE Keen, "The Effect of Heat upon the Biological Value of Meat Protein," *Journal of Nutrition* 7, no. 4 (April 1934): 367–79.

10 E Miller, "Laboratory Analysis of Pet Food," Division of Regulatory Services, University of Kentucky, 1996; and G Aldrich, personal communication, 2012.

11 K O'Rourke, "Zoonotic Risks of Pets: How to Handle Questions," *Journal of the American Veterinary Medical Association* 220, no. 10 (May 15, 2002): 1439, 1442.

12 T Hackett and MR Lappin, "Prevalence of Enteric Pathogens in Dogs of North-Central Colorado," *Journal of the American Animal Hospital Association* 39, no. 1 (January–February 2003): 52–56.

13 S Sanchez, CL Hofacre, MD Lee, et al.,

"Animal Sources of Salmonellosis," *Journal of the American Veterinary Medical Association* 221, no. 4 (August 15, 2002): 492–97.

14 J Dahlinger, SL Marks, and DC Hirsh, "Prevalence and Identity of Translocating Bacteria in Healthy Dogs," *Journal of Veterinary Internal Medicine* 11, no. 6 (November–December 1997): 319–22.

15 KJ Genovese, RC Anderson, RB Harvey, and DJ Nisbet, "Competitive Exclusion Treatment Reduces the Mortality and Fecal Shedding Associated with Enterotoxigenic *Escherichia coli* Infection in Nursery-Raised Neonatal Pigs," *Canadian Journal of Veterinary Research* 64, no. 4 (October 2000): 204–7.

16 E van Duijkeren and D Houwers, "Salmonella enteritis in Dogs, not Relevant? *Tijdschrift voor Diergeneeskund* 127, no. 23 (December 1, 2002): 716–17; MD Willard, B Sugarman, and RD Walker, "Gastrointestinal Zoonoses," *Veterinary Clinics of North America: Small Animal Practice* 17, no. 1 (January 1987): 145–78; RD Warner, "Occurrence and Impact of Zoonoses in Pet Dogs and Cats at U.S. Air Force Bases," *American Journal of Public Health* 74, no. 11 (November 1984):

1239–43; J Santamaria and GA Toranzos, "Enteric Pathogens and Soil: A Short Review," *International Journal of Microbiology* 6, no. 1 (March 2003): 5–9.

17 American Association of Feed Control Officers, *Official Publication,* 2013 (West Lafayette, Indiana: AAFCO, 2013): 135–41.

18 USDA National Nutrient Database for Standard Reference, http://ndb.nal.usda.gov.

19 ES Dierenfeld, HL Alcorn, and KL Jacobsen, "Nutrient Composition of Whole Vertebrate Prey (Excluding Fish) Fed in Zoos," USDA, 2002, http://www.nal.usda.gov/awic/zoo/WholePreyFinal02May29.pdf.

20 CA Daley, A Abbott, PS Doyle, et al., "A Review of Fatty Acid Profiles and Antioxidant Content in Grass-Fed and Grain-Fed Beef," *Nutrition Journal* 9 (2010): 10.

21 LM Freeman and KE Michel, "Evaluation of Raw Food Diets for Dogs," *Journal of the American Veterinary Medical Association* 218, no. 5 (2001): 705–9.

22 J Hofve, "Bad Science," *Whole Dog Journal* 4, no. 7 (July 2001): 12–13.

23 DA Fagan and MS Edwards, "Influence of Diet Consistency on Periodontal Dis-

ease in Captive Carnivores," http://www
.colyerinstitute.org/research/diet_consist
ency.htm.

24 MG Brown and JF Park, "Dental Calculus in Experimental Beagles," *Laboratory
Animal Care* 18, no. 5 (1968): 527–35.

25 ADJ Watson, "Diet and Periodontal
Disease in Dogs and Cats," *Australian
Veterinary Journal* 71 (1994): 313–18.

26 F Colyer, "Dental Disease in Animals,"
British Dental Journal 82 (1947): 31–35.

27 JAW Dollar, *Dollar's Veterinary Surgery:
General, Operative and Regional,* 4th ed.
(London: Baillière, Tindall, and Cox,
1950).

28 DA Crossley and S Penman, eds, Manual
of Small Animal Dentistry, 2nd ed. (Chel-
tenham: British Small Animal Veterinary
Association, 1995).

Chapter 10

1 A Atanda Jr., SA Shah, and K O'Brien,
"Osteochondrosis: Common Causes of
Pain in Growing Bones," *American Family
Physician* 83, no. 3 (February 1, 2011):
285–91.

2 RI Krontvelt, "Environmental Factors
Can Affect the Incidence of Hip Dysplasia in Dogs," Norwegian School of Veteri-

nary Science, March 15, 2012, http://www
.veths.no/en/Home/News/News-stories/A-
number-of-environmental-factors-can-
affect-the-incidence-of-hip-dysplasia-in-
dogs.

3 V Hart, P Nováková, EP Malkemper et
al., "Dogs Are Sensitive to Small Varia-
tions of the Earth's Magnetic Field." *Fron-
tiers in Zoology* 10, no. 80 (2013).

4 V Srinivasan, DW Spence, SR Pandi-
Perumal, et al., "Therapeutic Actions of
Melatonin in Cancer: Possible Mechanisms," *Integrated Cancer Therapies* 7, no.
3 (September 2008): 189–203, http://www
.umm.edu/altmed/articles/melatonin-
000315.htm#ixzz2OOIKZqAD.

5 LR Kogan, R Schoenfeld-Tacher, and AA
Simon, "Dogs Are Calmer with Classical
Music: Behavioral Effects of Auditory
Stimulation on Kenneled Dogs," *Journal
of Veterinary Behav*ior 7 (2012): 268–75.

6 "Acoustics: Standard Tuning Frequency
(Standard Musical Pitch)," International
Organization for Standardization 16
(1975), http://www.iso.org/iso/iso_cata
logue/catalogue_tc/catalogue_detail.htm?
csnumber=3601.

1 PS So, Y Jiang, and Y Qin, "Touch Therapies for Pain Relief in Adults," *Cochrane Database System Review* 4 (October 8, 2008): CD006535.

2 R Gallob, "Reiki: A Supportive Therapy in Nursing Practice and Self-Care for Nurses," *Journal of the New York State Nurses Association* 34, no. 1 (Spring–Summer 2003): 9–13.

3 A Kundu, R Dolan-Oves, MA Dimmers, et al., "Reiki Training for Caregivers of Hospitalized Pediatric Patients: A Pilot Program," *Complementary Therapies in Clinical Practices* 19, no. 1 (February 2013): 50–54, doi: 10.1016/j.ctcp.2012 .08.001.

4 SC Cuthbert and GJ Goodheart Jr., "On the Reliability and Validity of Manual Muscle Testing: A Literature Review," *Chiropractic and Osteopathy* 15 (March 6, 2007): 4.

5 P Hellyer, I Rodan, J Brunt, et al., "AAHA/AAFP Pain Management Guidelines for Dogs and Cats," *Journal of the American Animal Hospital Association* 43 (2007): 235–48.

6 K Lenger, "Homeopathic Potencies Iden-

tified by a New Magnetic Resonance Method: Homeopathy — an Energetic Medicine," *Subtle Energies and Energy Medicine: ISSSEEM Journal* 15, no. 3 (2004): 225–43.

Appendix A

1 DC Rule, KS Broughton, SM Shellito, et al., "Comparison of Muscle Fatty Acid Profiles and Cholesterol Concentrations of Bison, Beef Cattle, Elk, and Chicken," *Journal of Animal Science* 80 (2002): 1202–11.
2 RA Hansen, MA Harris, GE Pluhar, et al., "Fish Oil Decreases Matrix Metallo-proteinases in Knee Synovia of Dogs with Inflammatory Joint Disease," *Journal of Nutrition and Biochemistry* 19, no. 2 (February 19, 2008): 101–8.
3 J Leemans, C Cambier, T Chandler, et al., "Prophylactic Effects of Omega-3 Polyunsaturated Fatty Acids and Luteolin on Airway Hyperresponsiveness and In-flammation in Cats with Experimentally-Induced Asthma," *Veterinary Journal* 184, no. 1 (2010): 111–14, http://europepmc.org/abstract/MED/19231257/reload=0; jsessionid=tf9 wHojcEG37yTXo9fmA .30.

4 SA Brown, "Oxidative Stress and Chronic Kidney Disease," *Veterinary Clinics of North America: Small Animal Practice* 38, no. 1 (January 2008): 157–66, vi.

5 DP Laflamme, "Understanding and Managing Obesity in Dogs and Cats," *Veterinary Clinics of North America: Small Animal Practice* 36, no. 6 (November 2006): 1283–95, vii.

6 GE Billman, "A Comprehensive Review and Analysis of 25 Years of Data from an In Vivo Canine Model of Sudden Cardiac Death: Implications for Future Anti-Arrhythmic Drug Development," *Pharmacology and Therapeutics* 111, no. 3 (September 2006): 808–35.

7 P Roudebush, DJ Davenport, and BJ Novotny, "The Use of Nutraceuticals in Cancer Therapy," *Veterinary Clinics of North America: Small Animal Practice* 34, no. 1 (January 2004): 249–69, viii.

8 NW Milgram, E Head, CW Cotman, et al., "Age Dependent Cognitive Dysfunction in Canines: Dietary Intervention," in *Proceedings of the Third International Congress of Veterinary Behavioural Medicine*, edited by KL Overall, DS Mills, SE Heath, and D Horwitz (Wheathampstead, UK: Universities Federation for Animal Wel-

fare, 2001), 53–57.

9 S Re, M Zanoletti, and E Emanuele, "Aggressive Dogs Are Characterized by Low Omega-3 Polyunsaturated Fatty Acid Status," *Veterinary Research Communications* 32, no. 3 (March 2008): 225–30.

10 RA Hites, JA Foran, and DO Carpenter, "Global Assessment of Organic Contaminants in Farmed Salmon," *Science* 303, no. 5655 (January 9, 2004): 226–29, doi: 0.1126/science.1091447.

11 U.S. Fish and Wildlife Service, "Salmon of the West: What's the Difference between Wild and Hatchery Salmon?," http://www.fws.gov/salmonofthewest/Wild.htm.

12 RC Johnson, PK Weber, JD Wikert, et al., "Managed Metapopulations: Do Salmon Hatchery 'Sources' Lead to In-River 'Sinks' in Conservation?," *PLoS ONE* 7, no. 2 (2012): e28880, doi:10.1371/journal.pone.0028880.

13 P Greenberg, "A Fish Oil Story," *New York Times,* December 15, 2009, http://www.nytimes.com/2009/12/16/opinion/16greenberg.html/?_r=0.

14 Q Schiermeier, "Ecologists Fear Antarctic Krill Crisis," *Nature* 467, no. 15 (September 2010), http://www.nature.com/news/2010/100901/full/467015a.html.

15 TL Bierer and LM Bui, "Improvement

of Arthritic Signs in Dogs Fed Green-Lipped Mussel (*Perna canaliculus*)," *Journal of Nutrition* 132, no. 6, suppl. 2 (June 2002): 1634S–36S.

Appendix B

1 NG Robinson, "Problems with Raw Meat Diets," Colorado State University, 2007, http://csuvets.colostate.edu/pain/Articles pdf/Problems%20with%20Raw%20Meat .pdf.

2 DJ Joffe and DP Schlesinger, "Preliminary Assessment of the Risk of *Salmonella* Infection in Dogs Fed Raw Chicken Diets," *Canadian Veterinary Journal* 43, no. 6 (June 2002): 441–42.

3 K Hoelzer, AIM Switt, M Wiedmann, "Animal Contact as a Source of Human Non-Typhoidal Salmonellosis," *Veterinary Research* 42 (2011): 34.

4 R Finley, R Reid-Smith, JS Weese, et al., "Human Health Implications of *Salmonella*-Contaminated Natural Pet Treats and Raw Pet Food," *Clinical Infectious Diseases* 42 (2006): 686–91.

5 S Sanchez, CL Hofacre, MD Lee, et al., "Animal Sources of Salmonellosis," *Journal of the American Veterinary Medicine Association* 221, no. 4 (August 15, 2002):

492–97.

6 DP Laflamme, SK Abood, AJ Fascetti, et al., "Pet Feeding Practices of Dog and Cat Owners in the United States and Australia," *Journal of the American Veterinary Medicine Association* 2332, no. 5 (March 1, 2008): 687–94.

7 K O'Rourke, "Zoonotic Risks of Pets: How to Handle Questions," *Journal of the American Veterinary Medicine Association* 220, no. 10 (May 15, 2002): 1439–42.

8 DD Hancock, "Public Health Concerns Associated with Feeding Raw Meat Diets to Dogs," *Journal of the American Veterinary Medicine Association* 219 (2001): 1222–25.

9 MB Skirrow, "*Campylobacter enteritis* in Dogs and Cats: A 'New' Zoonosis," *Veterinary Research Communications* 5, no. 1 (September 5, 1981): 13–19.

10 DJ Wilson, E Gabriel, AJ Leatherbarrow, et al., "Tracing the Source of Campylobacteriosis," *PLoS Genetics* 4, no. 9 (September 2008): e1000203.

11 K Bischoff and WK Rumbeiha, "Pet Food Recalls and Pet Food Contaminants in Small Animals," *Veterinary Clinics of North America: Small Animal Practice* 42, no. 2 (March 2012): 237–50.

12 JL Jones, V Dargelas, J Roberts, et al., "Risk Factors for *Toxoplasma gondii* Infection in the United States," *Clinical Infectious Diseases* 49, no. 6 (September 15, 2009): 878–84.

13 AL Salb, HW Barkema, BT Elkin, et al., "Dogs as Sources and Sentinels of Parasites in Humans and Wildlife, Northern Canada," *Emerging Infectious Diseases* 14, no. 1 (January 2008), http://wwwnc.cdc.gov/eid/article/14/1/07-1113.htm.

14 JA Barsanti, M Walser, CL Hatheway, et al., "Type C Botulism in American Foxhounds," *Journal of the American Veterinary Medicine Association* 172, no. 7 (April 1, 1978): 809–13.

15 A Uriarte, J-L Thibaud, and S Blot, "Botulism in 2 Urban Dogs," *Canadian Veterinary Journal* 51, no. 10 (October 2010): 1139–42.

16 JP Dubey, G Schares, and LM Ortega-Mora, "Epidemiology and Control of Neosporosis and *Neospora caninum*," *Clinical Microbiology Review* 20, no. 2 (April 2007): 323–67, doi: 10.1128/CMR.000 31-06 PMCID: PMC1865591.

17 J Lenz, D Joffe, M Kauffman, et al., "Perceptions, Practices, and Consequences Associated with Foodborne

Pathogens and the Feeding of Raw Meat to Dogs," *Canadian Veterinary Journal* 50, no. 6 (June 2009): 637–43.

18 TC Smith, MJ Male, AL Harper, et al., "Methicillin-Resistant *Staphylococcus aureus* (MRSA) Strain ST398 Is Present in Midwestern U.S. Swine and Swine Workers," *PLoS ONE* 4, no. 1: e4258, doi:10.1371/journal.pone.0004258, http://www.plosone.org/article/info:doi/10.1371/journal.pone.0004258.

19 MB Boost, MM O'Donoghue, and A James, "Prevalence of *Staphylococcus aureus* Carriage among Dogs and Their Owners," *Epidemiology and Infection* 136, no. 7 (July 2008): 953–64.

20 J Cullor, University of California at Davis, Veterinary Medical Teaching and Research Center, Tulare, California, unpublished data and personal communications, 1999–2000.

21 CE Greene, "Yersiniosis," in *Infectious Diseases of the Dog and Cat,* 3rd ed. (St. Louis, Missouri: WB Saunders, 2007), 361–62.

22 RF Kahrs, DN Holmes, and GC Poppensiek, "Diseases Transmitted from Pets to Man: An Evolving Concern for Veterinarians," *Cornell Veterinarian* 68, no. 4 (October 1978): 442–59.

23 AN Beloshapka, LM Duclos, BM Vester Boler, et al., "Effects of Inulin or Yeast Cell-Wall Extract on Nutrient Digestibility, Fecal Fermentative Endproduct Concentrations, and Blood Metabolite Concentrations in Adult Dogs Fed Raw Meat-Based Diets," *American Journal of Veterinary Research* 73, no. 7 (July 2012): 1016–23; SM Murray, AR Patil, GC Fahey, et al., "Raw and Rendered Animal By-Products as Ingredients in Dog Diets," *Journal of Animal Science* 75 (1997): 2497–505; KR Kerr, BM Vester Boler, CL Morris, et al., "Apparent Total Tract Energy and Macronutrient Digestibility and Fecal Fermentative End-Product Concentrations of Domestic Cats Fed Extruded, Raw Beef-Based, and Cooked Beef-Based Diets," *Journal of Animal Science* 90, no. 2 (February 2012): 515–22; and BM Vester, SL Burke, KJ Liu, et al., "Influence of Feeding Raw or Extruded Feline Diets on Nutrient Digestibility and Nitrogen Metabolism of African Wildcats (*Felis lybica*)," *Zoology and Biology* 29, no. 6 (November–December 2010): 676–86.

24 CA Kirk, personal communication.

GLOSSARY

Adaptogen: A substance that increases vital energy, helps the body adapt to stress, and restores functional balance to all organs and systems.

Adjuvants: Substances used in vaccines that stimulate inflammation and increase the immune response. An adjuvanted vaccine usually contains a killed virus or organism.

Adrenaline: A hormone released by the adrenal glands in response to a sudden fright.

Allopathic: Pertaining to conventional medicine, also commonly referred to as Western medicine.

Alterative: A substance that gradually restores overall health.

Analgesic: Providing relief from pain.

Antiaging: Preventing or delaying degenerative changes associated with increasing age.

Antibodies: The blood proteins manufactured by the immune system *B-lymphocytes* that attack and destroy invading organisms; antibody production is the goal of vaccination.

Antiemetic: A substance that inhibits vomiting.

Antineoplastic: A substance that inhibits tumor growth.

Antioxidant: A substance that destroys *oxygen free radicals.*

Aromatherapy: The use of scent from essential oils to treat mental and physical conditions.

Astromedicine: A branch of astrology that studies the tendencies of a person or an animal toward health and sickness, indicating the periods in which they are most vulnerable to disease.

Aura: A colorful energetic "halo" all around the body; also called the etheric double.

Autoantibodies: Antibodies that react against the body's own tissues.

Autoimmune: A condition in which antibodies react to and destroy the body's own tissues. Examples of such conditions include lupus, canine hypothyroidism, and immune-mediated hemolytic anemia.

Autonomic nervous system: The "involuntary" part of the peripheral nervous system (outside the brain and spinal cord) that controls organ functions such as heart rate, breathing, and digestion.

Beneficial nematodes: Beneficial, predatory worms that eat flea eggs and help control flea populations outdoors.

Bioavailability: The degree to which a food or other substance is digested, absorbed into the bloodstream, and used by the body.

Bioidentical hormones: Products created in a laboratory by altering compounds derived from naturally occurring plant products; typically come in the form of creams or gels.

Biomimicry: A new science that studies nature's models and then uses these designs and processes to solve human problems.

Bioresonance: The quality of harmony between two living beings. In holistic healing, the term is used to describe a multitude of techniques and devices used to diagnose and/or treat illnesses through energy fields.

B-lymphocytes: White blood cells that are part of the immune system; when stimulated, they produce *antibodies.*

Brachycephalic: A congenital malformation of the skull in which premature closure of the coronal suture results in excessive lateral growth of the head, giving it a short, broad appearance.

Capillary: The tiniest blood vessels that directly contact the cells.

Carbohydrate (carb): A macronutrient. An organic molecule, such as sugar, starch, or fiber, made of carbon, hydrogen, and oxygen.

Carcinogen: A cancer-causing chemical or other agent.

Chakra: One of the seven main energetic centers of the body.

Chromosome: A packet of tightly coiled *DNA* that contains all the genetic material of the organism. Humans have 46 chromosomes (23 pairs); dogs and wolves have 78 chromosomes (39 pairs).

Circadian: Having a biological rhythm with a 24-hour light-dark pattern.

Colostrum: A thin yellowish fluid secreted by the mammary glands of female mammals at the time of parturition that is rich in antibodies and minerals and precedes the production of true milk.

Cortisol: A hormone made by the adrenal glands that mediates the chronic stress response. It suppresses the immune system and thyroid function and impairs bone and tissue repair.

Darwinian: Related to Charles Darwin (1809–1882) or the principles of his theory of evolution, such as "survival of the fittest" and "evolution proceeds by chance mutation."

Denature: (1) To distort or alter the fundamental structure or nature of a substance. For example, a denatured protein has lost its natural shape and can no longer perform its function. Proteins can become denatured due to extreme conditions, such as high heat or chemical processing. Denatured proteins are thought to be more allergenic than normal proteins. (2) To make unnatural by adding an inedible substance; some foods are purposely adulterated during processing to make them unfit for human consumption but acceptable for other uses, such as pet food. The most common methods of denaturing animal products is with dye or charcoal.

Dentition: The arrangement, type, and number of an animal's teeth. For example, a dog's dentition consists of 42 teeth: 12 incisors, 4 canines (fangs), 16 premolars, and 10 molars.

Detoxification: A natural phase of the healing process that occurs when changes in diet and environment remove the residue and effects of drugs, vaccines, anesthesia, chemicals, processed pet food, and infectious agents. During detoxification, things may seem to get worse for a time, even though the body is actually moving forward to restore health and balance.

Diuretic: Promoting water loss through urine.

DNA (deoxyribonucleic acid): A molecule with a double helix structure that contains genes and directs the growth and function of living organisms. Pairs of nucleic acids wrap in a double strand around proteins called histones.

Electromagnetic fields (EMFs): All plants and animals operate by tiny electrochemical pulses at about the same frequency as the energy field here on the earth. Cell phones, computers, televisions, and other appliances all produce toxic EMFs.

Emotional Freedom Techniques: A technique of tapping on acupuncture *meridians* to help release emotional trauma or heal physical ailments.

Endocrine: Producing hormones; usually refers to glands such as the thyroid or pancreas that secrete hormones into the blood for distribution.

Endogenous: Made by or within the body.

Epigenetics: Heritable changes in the way

genes are expressed that do not involve replication of *DNA.*

Epigenome: The molecular tags covering each strand of *DNA* that control which genes are active. (The prefix *epi-* means "above.")

Euthanasia: Literally, "good death"; used to describe the humane killing of an animal. In pets, this is typically done through injection of an overdose of barbiturates.

Excipient-free supplements: Supplements that do not contain additives or fillers, such as magnesium stearate, stearic acid, cellulose, etc.

Exogenous: Something from outside the body.

Fat, fatty acid: Fat is a macronutrient; fatty acids are the building blocks of fat. Each fat molecule (also called a triglyceride) is made up of three fatty acid chains attached to a glycerol molecule.

Febrifuge: A substance that reduces *fever.*

Fecal transplant: The introduction of feces from a healthy individual into the rectum of the patient in order to reestablish a normal bacterial population.

Fever: A body temperature above the canine normal of 101.5°F. Fever can be caused by stress, infection, immune system dysfunction (autoimmune disease), or cancer.

Fiber: An indigestible complex carbohydrate made exclusively by plants.

Flower essences (remedies): Specially prepared energetic extracts of flowers and other substances that act as gentle catalysts to alleviate stress and restore emotional balance.

Glycemic index: A measurement of how high and how fast a particular carbohydrate raises blood sugar levels.

Glycogen: The storage form of glucose in the liver and muscles.

Health: Not just the absence of symptoms but also an overall feeling of well-being and vitality.

Hemostatic: A substance that stops bleeding.

Hepatic: Pertaining to the liver.

Herd immunity: The establishment of immunity in a large percentage of animals in a population so that if a disease does break out, there will not be enough susceptible animals to sustain an epidemic. The idea was first developed for livestock.

Holistic: A philosophy of well-being that considers the physical, mental, emotional, and spiritual aspects of life as closely interconnected and balanced. A holistic approach to veterinary medicine takes into account the breed, lifestyle, diet, activity level, and social environment as well as the medical history and current symptoms.

Homeopathy: A system of healing developed by Samuel Hahnemann, a German medical doctor, in the late 18th century.

Homeostasis: The equilibrium (balance) maintained by an organism through constant adjustment of its internal physiological processes.

Horizontal transmission: The transfer of a pathogen from an infected animal to an unexposed animal, independent of the parental relationship of those individuals.

Hot spot (lick granuloma): A defined area where a dog constantly licks, causing hair loss, redness, swelling, and irritation that often progresses to a moist open wound. May be caused by itchiness, pain in the underlying tissues, or nerve trauma.

Immunosenescence: The slow deterioration of the immune system as a result of the aging process.

Inoculate: To physically introduce or inject a microorganism, such as with a vaccine, or to introduce or inject friendly bacteria into the gastrointestinal tract, as in probiotic therapy or fecal transplant.

Lick granuloma: See *hot spot*.

Macronutrient: One of three major classes

of nutrients: protein, fat, and carbohydrate.

Malocclusion: A mismatch between the upper and lower teeth; an abnormal bite.

Matrix: The area between cells; also called ground substance. Blood and lymph vessels and nerves run through the matrix; oxygen and nutrients must diffuse across the matrix to reach cells; carbon dioxide and cellular waste products move back across the matrix to be removed.

Melatonin: A hormone produced by the pineal gland that regulates the sleeping and waking cycles, among other processes. It is also a very strong antioxidant. Deficient levels have been associated with several disorders, including cancer.

Meme: An idea that spreads from person to person or acts as a unit for carrying cultural ideas, symbols, or practices, via writing, speech, gestures, rituals, or other phenomena.

Meridians: A system of interconnected pathways through which the energy (*qi*) of the body flows. Hundreds of acupuncture points (acupoints) occur along these pathways.

Microbe: Any microscopic organism such as a bacterium, fungus, or virus.

Microbiome: The totality of organisms that

naturally inhabit the body.

Negative ions: Negatively charged particles that are experienced during rain, at the seashore, near a waterfall, or in a forest. (In contrast, positive ions are found more in desert habitats and where there is a lot of concrete.)

Nematode: Roundworm.

Neuter: Surgical sterilization; removal of the male reproductive glands (testes). Also referred to as desexing and/or altering.

Nonverbal communication: A skill that many believe all life-forms shared before we had language, allowing us to communicate among ourselves and with animals.

Nosodes: Homeopathically prepared remedies made from disease material, such as tissues, discharges, or secretions. Nosodes can be used to treat infectious diseases and are sometimes utilized as a part of a prevention protocol in much the same way as vaccines are.

Nutraceuticals: Nutritional supplementation for a specific purpose, such as glucosamine and methylsulfonylmethane (MSM) for arthritis.

Operant conditioning: A stimulus-response behavior modification (training) method for dogs based on the way all animals learn.

Osteochondrosis: A painful skeletal disorder in growing animals.

Overt: Visible or obvious to an observer.

Oxidation: In the body, the process of using oxygen to create energy. This process occurs in the mitochondria, small organs (organelles) within each cell.

Oxygen free radicals (reactive oxygen species): Highly chemically reactive molecules that contain oxygen.

Parasympathetic nervous system: The part of the autonomic nervous system that includes cranial nerves and lower spinal nerves, which are involved in the sensations of taste and smell and help regulate blood oxygen and carbon dioxide levels and other functions.

Parturition: Delivery of offspring; birth.

Pathogen: Any disease-causing organism.

Pathogenic: Disease-causing.

Pathological: Abnormal; unhealthy; causing or contributing to disease.

Peptide, polypeptide: A peptide is a short chain of amino acids; a polypeptide is a longer chain of peptides that makes up all or part of a protein.

Periodontitis: Inflammation of the periodontium caused by bacteria that infect the roots of teeth and the surrounding gum crevices.

pH: A measurement of how acid or alkaline a substance is. Water has a neutral pH of 7.0; less than 7.0 is acidic, and over 7.0 is alkaline. Normal dog urine pH ranges between 5.5 and 7.0. A dog eating a high-protein meat-based diet will have a lower urine pH than a dog eating dry food.

Plasma cells: Tiny but high-powered factories that produce antibodies against a particular disease.

Pottenger's Cats: A study conducted between 1932 and 1942 by Francis M. Pottenger Jr., MD, over many generations of cats to determine the effects of cooking their food on their health.

Poultice: A moist, hot herbal pack applied topically that can be used, for instance, to treat a bite wound or an abscess.

Protein: A macronutrient made up of chains of amino acids and *polypeptides.*

Pulsed electromagnetic field therapy (PEMF): Using electrical energy to direct a series of magnetic pulses through injured tissue whereby each pulse induces a tiny electrical signal that stimulates cellular repair.

Qi (Chi): In traditional Chinese medicine,

the vital life force present in all living beings.

Reiki: A system of hands-on energy healing developed in Japan from techniques used in ancient Asian cultures.

Renal: Pertaining to the kidneys.

Rendering: A process of slow cooking (boiling) for many hours to separate the fat and kill pathogens such as bacteria, viruses, and parasites.

Spay: Surgical sterilization; removal of the reproductive organs (desexing) of the female dog; technically called ovariohysterectomy.

Species-specific diet: The diet an animal would eat in its natural habitat.

Specific gravity: A measurement of urine concentration. Dogs eating dry food tend to have highly concentrated urine (up to 1.050), while dogs eating wet food produce a more diluted urine (closer to 1.015).

Spirochetal bacteria: Any of a family of spiral- or coil-shaped bacteria, such as the *Borrelia* bacteria that causes Lyme disease.

Stenosis: A narrowing or stricture of a passage or vessel.

Subluxation: A term used in chiropractic medicine for small displacements or dislocations of the vertebrae or other joints. A luxation is a complete dislocation; a sub-luxation is less dramatic.

Suppression: In homeopathy, this term is used to explain how a treatment can get rid of specific symptoms, but may simultaneously drive the disease into other channels by denying the body's expression of the original disease. Suppressive medicines are often named with the prefix *anti-:* antibiotics, antipyretics, anti-inflammatories, etc.

Symbiotic: Living in symbiosis or having an interdependent relationship. Many people feel the relationship between humans and dogs is symbiotic.

Sympathetic nervous system: A branch of the autonomic nervous system; best known for the "fight or flight" response in animals.

Taurine deficiency: Studies suggest that consumption of certain commercial pet foods may be associated with low blood or plasma taurine concentrations and dilated cardiomyopathy.

Taxonomy: The formal system of classifying and naming organisms.

Terrain: The cells and tissues of the body.

Therapeutic touch: An energy therapy that promotes healing and reduces pain by the simple act of placing the human hand(s) on or near a human or animal patient. This may allow the practitioner to detect energy imbalances in the patient and impart a healing response.

Thermoregulation: The internal temperature control system of warm-blooded animals.

Vaccination: Inoculation with a vaccine in order to induce an immunological response to a particular disease.

Vaccinosis: In homeopathic medicine, a chronic condition with multiple symptoms.

Vector: A carrier of disease, such as a rodent, tick, or mosquito.

Vertebrae: The bones of the spine (backbone).

Vertical transmission: Passage of a disease-causing agent (pathogen) from mother to baby during the period immediately before and after birth.

Whole food supplements: Nutrients as they are found in a given food, as opposed to when you isolate a nutrient or vitamin from the food complex within which it is naturally found.

Wobbler syndrome: A disorder of the cervical (neck) vertebrae and spinal cord that manifests as an unsteady or wobbly gait, especially in the hind legs.

RESOURCES

ASSOCIATIONS, ORGANIZATIONS, AND SERVICES

Academy of Veterinary Homeopathy
866-652-1590
www.theavh.org
Certification course for veterinary homeopathy

AltVetMed: Complementary and Alternative Veterinary Medicine
www.altvetmed.org

American Academy of Veterinary Acupuncture
800-632-9911
www.aava.org

American Holistic Veterinary Medical Association
410-569-0795

www.ahvma.org
Publishes the Journal of the American
Holistic Veterinary Medical Association
and has a practitioner directory at www
.ahvma.org/Widgets/FindVet.html

American Institute of Homeopathy
888-445-9988
www.homeopathyusa.org
Publishes the Journal of the American
Institute of Homeopathy

American Veterinary Chiropractic
* Association*
918-784-2231
www.animalchiropractic.org
Certification course for veterinary chiropractic

Animal Talk
* Penelope Smith*
www.animaltalk.net/
Directory of professional animal com-
municators

ASPCA Animal Poison Control Center
888-426-4435
www.aspca.org/pet-care/animal-poison-
  control
Animal poison-related emergency information, 24/7

*Association of British Veterinary
  Acupuncturists*
www.abva.co.uk

*Australian Veterinary Chiropractic
  Association*
www.chirovet.com.au

Bio-Integral Resource Center
510-524-2567
www.birc.org

*British Association of Homeopathic
  Veterinary Surgeons*
www.bahvs.com

Cal Pet Crematory
818-983-2313, 323-875-0633,
  310-278-0633
www.calpet.com
The dog's remains can be shipped frozen
using overnight mail. Extremely reliable
group that ensures you get your dog's
ashes back.

Chi Institute
800-891-1986
Certification courses for veterinary acupuncture
www.tcvm.com

Energetic Medicine Research
www.energetic-medicine.net (info)
www.energetic-healing.com (store)

Flower Essence Society
800-736-9222
www.flowersociety.org
Research on flower essences and professional association.

Gary Craig
  Emotional Freedom Technique
www.emofree.com
Founder of the Emotional Freedom Technique, which combines mind-body medicine and tapping; directory of certified professional EFT practitioners

Grief Recovery Institute
800-445-4808
www.grief-recovery.com

International Foundation for Nutrition and Health
858-488-8932
www.ifnh.org

International Veterinary Acupuncture Society
970-266-0666

www.ivas.org
Certification course for veterinary acupuncture

National Animal Supplement Council
760-751-3360
www.nasc.cc
Nonprofit industry group dedicated to protecting and enhancing the health of companion animals and horses; certifies products meeting its rigorous standards

National United Professional Association
  of Trained Homeopaths (Canada)
519-748-2224
www.nupath.org

Natural Rearing Breeders Directory
www.nrbreeders.homestead.com

Price-Pottenger Nutrition Foundation
800-366-3748
619-462-7600
www.ppnf.org
A nonprofit education organization dedicated to the promotion of enhanced health through an awareness of ecology, lifestyle, and healthy food production for good nutrition. Catalog of books, pamphlets, and tapes available.

Richard Pitcairn, DVM, PhD
  Animal Natural Health Center
www.drpitcairn.com
Author and lecturer; online referral
directory for veterinary homeopaths.

Veterinary Botanical Medical Association
www.vbma.org
Certification courses for veterinary herbalism and veterinary herbalism educator

Veterinary Institute of Integrative Medicine
303-277-8227
www.viim.org

Washington Animal Disease Diagnostic
  Lab
509-335-9696
www.vetmed.wsu.edu/depts_waddl/
Provides necropsy services

Weston A. Price Foundation
202-363-4394
www.westonaprice.org
Provides nutrition education information

W. Jean Dodds, DVM
938 Stanford Street
Santa Monica, CA 90403

310-828-4804
www.hemopet.org
Founder and president of Hemopet, co-
ordinator of the Rabies Challenge Fund

BOOKS

Aromatherapy, Flower Essences, and Herbs

Bell, Kristen Leigh. *Holistic Aromatherapy for Animals.* Findhorn, Scotland: Findhorn Press, 2002.

Grosjean, Nelly. *Veterinary Aromatherapy.* Saffron Walden, United Kingdom: C.W. Daniel Co, 2005. www.nellygrosjean.com.

The Sthitaprajna. *Sai Sanjeevini: A Healer's Guide.* New Delhi, India.www.saisanjeevini.org.

Wulff-Tilford, Mary, and Gregory Tilford. *All You Ever Wanted to Know about Herbs for Pets.* Irvine, CA: BowTie Press, 2001.

Behavior and Training

Pryor, Karen. *Clicker Training.* Waltham, PA: Sunshine Books, 2003. www.clickertraining.com.

McConnell, Patricia B. and Aimee M. Moore. *Family Friendly Dog Training: A Six-*

Week Program for You and Your Dog. Black Earth, WI: Dog's Best Friend, 2006. www .patriciamcconnell.com.

Yin, Sophia DVM. *How to Behave So Your Dog Behaves.* Neptune, NJ: THF Publications, 2010.

This and other books, videos, DVDs, and training tools are available at www .drsophiayin.com

Holistic Health Care

Chambreau, Christina. *Healthy Animal's Journal: What You Can Do to Have Your Dog or Cat Live a Long and Healthy Life.* Sparks, MD: TRO Productions, 2003. www.christinachambreau.com.

Dog, Chiclet T. and Jan Rasmusen. *Scared Poopless.* Rancho Santa Fe, CA: dogs4dogs, 2006. www.dogs4dogs.com.

Fox, Michael W. *The Healing Touch: The Proven Massage Program for Dogs.* New York: Newmarket Press, 2004, revised edition. www.doctormwfox.org.

Fulton, Elizabeth, and Kathleen Prasad. *Animal Reiki.* Berkeley, CA: Ulysses Press, 2006. www.animalreikisource.com.

Goldstein, Martin. *The Nature of Animal Healing: The Definitive Holistic Medicine Guide to Caring for Your Dog and Cat.* New

518

York: Random House, 2009.

Hamilton, Don. *Homeopathic Care for Cats and Dogs: Small Doses for Small Animals.* Berkeley, CA: North Atlantic Books, 2005. www.ppnf.org.

Hofve, Jean. *What Dogs Should Eat.* Denver, CO: Vetwise Publishing, 2012. www.little bigcat.com.

Pottenger, Francis M., Jr. *Pottenger's Cats: A Study in Nutrition.* La Mesa, CA: Lemon Grove, 1995.

Schwartz, Cheryl. *Four Paws, Five Directions: A Guide to Chinese Medicine for Cats and Dogs.* Berkeley, CA: Celestial Arts, 1996.

Shojai, Amy. *ComPETability: Solving Behavior Problems In Your Multi-Dog Household.* FurryMuse Publications, 2012.

Tellington-Jones, Linda. *Getting in TTouch with Your Dog: A Gentle Approach to Influencing Behavior, Health, and Performance.* North Pomfret, VT: Trafalgar Square Press, 2003. www.ttouch.com.

Yarnall, Celeste. *Natural Dog Care: A Complete Guide to Holistic Health Care for Dogs.* Edison, NJ: Castle, 2000. www.celestial pets.com.

Yarnall, Celeste and Jean Hofve, DVM. *The Complete Guide to Holistic Cat Care: An Il-*

lustrated Manual. Boston, MA: Quarry Books, 2009. http://tinyurl.com/24vhufm.

Zidonis, Nancy A., and Amy Snow. *Acu-Dog: A Guide to Canine Acupressure.* Larkspur, CO: Tallgrass Publishers, LLC, 2011. www.animalacupressure.com.

Zucker, Martin. *Veterinarians' Guide to Natural Remedies for Dogs: Safe and Effective Alternative Treatments and Healing Techniques from the Nations' Top Holistic Veterinarians.* New York: Crown (Random House), 2010.

Immunization and Vaccines

O'Driscoll, Catherine. *Shock to the System: The Facts about Animal Vaccination, Pet Food and How to Keep Your Pets Healthy.* Wenatchee, WA: Dogwise, 2005.

New Age, Quantum Healing, and Antiaging

Emoto, Masaru. *The Hidden Messages in Water.* New York: Atria Books/Simon & Schuster, 2011.

Lipton, Bruce H. *The Biology of Belief: Unleashing the Power of Consciousness, Matter and Miracles.* Santa Rosa, CA: Mountain Love/Elite Books, 2005.

Lipton, Bruce H., and Steve Bhaerman. *Spontaneous Evolution: Our Positive Future and a Way to Get There from Here.* Carlsbad, CA: Hay House, 2009.

McTaggart, Lynne. *The Field: The Quest for the Secret Force of the Universe.* New York: Harper, 2008.

Melody, A. *Love Is in the Earth: A Kaleidoscope of Crystals — The Reference Book Describing Metaphysical Properties of the Mineral Kingdom.* Richland, WA: Earth-Love Publishing House, 1995.

Perry, Wayne. *Sound Medicine: The Complete Guide to Healing with the Human Voice.* Franklin Lakes, NJ: New Page Books, 2007. www.wayneperry.com.

Wiley, T S., with Bent Formby. *Lights Out: Sugar, Sleep, and Survival.* New York: Simon and Schuster, 2000. www.thewiley protocol.com.

NONVERBAL COMMUNICATION

Boone, J. Allen. *Kinship with All Life.* New York: Harper One, 1979.

Lydecker, Beatrice. *Stories the Animals Tell Me.* New York: Harper & Row Publishers, 1979.

Schoen, Allen M. *Kindred Spirits.* New York: Broadway, 2001. www.drschoen.com.

Smith, Penelope. *Animal Talk: Interspecies Telepathic Communication.* Hillsboro, OR:

Beyond Words Publishing, 2008. www.animaltalk.net.

Solisti, Kate. *Conversations with Dog: An Uncommon Dogalog of Canine Wisdom.* Tulsa, OK: Council Oak Books, 2004. www.akinshipwithanimals.com.

Pet Loss

Congalton, David, and Charlotte Alexander. *When Your Pet Outlives You: Protecting Animal Companions after You Die.* Troutdale, OR: New Sage Press, 2002.

Smith, Penelope. *Animals in Spirit.* Hillsboro, OR: Beyond Words Publishing, 2008. www.animaltalk.net.

Stone, B. Cat. *The Cat in the Music Box: A Message from Pet Heaven.* Cat Box Press, 2013.

Pest Control

Olkowski, William, Sheila Dear, and Helga Olkowski. *Common Sense Pest Control: Least Toxic Solutions for Your Home, Garden, Pets and Community.* Newtown, CT: Taunton Press, 1991.

Sammons, Chip. *Flea Control: A Holistic and Humorous Approach.* Clackamas, OR: Holistic Pet Center, 1996.

Tvedten, Stephen. *Natural Mosquito Control: How to Get Rid of Mosquitoes Fast Without Toxic Chemicals or Insecticides* (Organic Pest Control). TCK Publishing, 2013.

EDUCATIONAL RESOURCES

College of Integrative Veterinary Therapies
www.civtedu.org
Courses on holistic and integrative therapies for lay and veterinary practitioners.

Lang Institute for Canine Massage
P.O. Box 2786
Loveland CO 80539-2786
877-669-3929
http://dogmassage.com

Linda Tellington-Jones
866-488-6824
505-455-2945
www.ttouch.com
Founder and instructor of the Tellington T-Touch method. Books, videos, and training available.

TVMED Corporation 2002
RAmEx Ars Medica
800-633-8271

310-826-4964
www.ramex.com/title.asp?id=9007
Video on theory and application of the
Bi-Digital O-Ring muscle test

HEALTH PRACTITIONERS

Professional Specialists

Carol Gurney
818-597-1154
www.animalcommunicator.net
Animal communicator and bodywork

Lydia Hiby
760-796-4304
www.lydiahiby.com
Animal communicator, analyst, and
author. Available for consultants, lec-
tures, and seminars.

William L. Inman, BS, DVM, CVCP
208-772-4360
www.vomtech.com
Teacher and lecturer. Developed the
Veterinary Orthopedic Manipulation
technique. Founder and head of the
International Association of Veterinary
Chiropractitioners

Laura Mignosa, NCCH
  Connecticut Institute of Herbal Studies
860-666-5064
www.ctherbschool.com
Nationally certified Chinese herbalist and director of the Connecticut Institute of Herbal Studies

Carol Pollard
303-694-7414
www.carolpollard.com
Animal communicator

Susanne Peach
303-926-5414
www.animaleze.com
EFT Practitioner for humans and animals

Wayne Perry
800-276-8634
323-655-7781
www.wayneperry.com
Founder and director of the Sound Therapy Center of Los Angeles, sound therapist

Kathleen Prasad
415-420-9783
www.animalreikisource.com
Reiki Master

Joan R. Ranquet
888-882-7208
425-788-3888
www.joanranquet.com
Animal communicator, author, and teacher

Kate Solisti
303-568-9048
www.akinshipwithanimals.com
Animal communicator and author; classes and one-on-one mentoring/ apprenticeships; nutritional consultations

The Tapping Solution
EFT training, videos, and resources
www.thetappingsolution.com

Laura Stinchfield
www.thepetpsychic.com
Animal communication

Celeste Yarnall, PhD
818-707-6331
www.celestialpets.com
Available for consultations regarding the fresh/raw food diet and supplementation, and alternative healing therapies for dogs and cats.

Veterinarians

Susan Beal, DVM
  Big Run Healing Arts
319 East Main Street, Box 555
Big Run, PA 15715
814-427-5004
Veterinary specialist in homeopathy, cranial sacral therapy, veterinary chiropractic. Available for telephone consultation.

Stephen Blake, DVM
858-566-3588
San Diego, CA 92131
www.thepetwhisperer.com

Bert H. Brooks, DVM and Melissa Brooks, BS
  Cache Creek Vet Service
15200 County Road 96B
Woodland, CA 95695
530-666-7322
www.cchvs.com
NAET, ETA, Harmonic Translation. Available for telephone consultation.

Christina Chambeau, DVM
908 Coldbottom Road
Sparks, MD 21152

410-771-4968
www.christinachambreau.com
www.healthyanimalsjournal.com
Academy of Veterinary Homeopathy founding member who teaches veterinary homeopathy for pet guardians and animal professionals. Available for telephone consultation.

Charles E. Loops, DVM
Route 2, Box 568
Pittsboro, NC 27312
919-542-0442
www.charlesloopsdvm.com
Available for telephone consultation on homeopathy, nosodes, and vaccination issues

Russell Swift, DVM
7154 North University Drive #86
Tamarac, FL 33321
877-239-3552
561-391-5615
www.therightremedy.com
Classical homeopath and veterinary chiropractor. Available for telephone consultation.

MEAT & DAIRY PRODUCTS

Harmony Farms
818-248-3068
www.harmonyfarmsca.com
A variety of raw meats, including chicken and turkey necks, as well as Celeste Yarnall's Carnivore Mix.

Organic Pastures
877-RAW-MILK
www.organicpastures.com
Raw organic beef, milk, cream, butter and cheese

NUTRITIONAL SUPPLEMENTS

Celestial Pets Natural Nutrition and Holistic Health Care
818-707-6331
www.celestialpets.com
Complete supplements for homemade pet diets, including Celestial Pets® Vita-Mineral Plus, Essential Fatty Acid Oil for Dogs, Canine Enzyme Supplement; as well as NanoVi Active Air, BEMER, Himalayan Crystal Salt, and much more; see website and/or call for information regarding clinical nutrition services and products mentioned throughout this book.

Geneflora

www.cycles-of-life.com/
  ProductGenefloraPets.html
Probiotic/enzyme combination products.
If you get human capsules, be sure you
dose appropriately for your pet's size.

Moxxor

www.moxxholisticvet.com(info)
www.holisticvet.moxxor.com/buy/
  (order)
New Zealand Green-lipped Mussel Oil
omega-3 supplement with super-
antioxidants

Hyalun Oral Hyaluronic Acid

866-318-8484
913-422-9395
www.hyalun.com
Hyaluronic acid joint supplement for
horses that is also suitable for pets

Only Natural Pet Store

888-937-6677
www.onlynaturalpet.com
Natural dog food, supplements, and pet
supplies. Save 15% on any single order
with coupon code PALEO.

Optimum Choices

866-305-2306

303-271-1649
www.optimumchoices.com
BioPreparation and BioSuperfood blue-green algae products special blend of spirulina and other algae selected for their easily digested polysaccharide cell wall, for pets and people.

Pets' Friend
800-868-1009
561-391-3397
www.mypetsfriend.com
Dr. Russell Swift's enzyme formulas (FloraZyme EFA and FloraZyme LP), Pet G.O. multiple glandular and organ concentrates, Celestial Pets VitaMineral Plus and feline enzyme supplements, Trace AniMinerals, PetiGreens, and other natural healing products

Protandim Canine
www.mylifevantage.com/lvhealth/
High potency herbal antioxidant as well as antioxidant and joint support (Distributed by Celestial Pets)

Salba Chia Seeds
Whole or ground chia seeds are a source of Omega-3 fatty acids, fiber, and micronutrients; Salba is certified non-

GMO and gluten-free. (Distributed by Celestial Pets)

PRODUCTS

Aromatherapy and Herbs

Grapefruit Seed Extract GSE®
Liquid concentrate from certified organically grown grapefruit with a myriad of uses. (Distributed by Celestial Pets)

Living Libations
  Aromatherapy Hydrosol Mists
www.livinglibations.com#a_aid=50ad
  905688dc5
Luxurious hydrosols in several varieties, including calming Bulgarian Lavender, energizing Red Clover Tea, and invigorating Sandalwood Vanilla

Ojibwa Tea of Life
www.ojibwatea.com
Organic and ethically-wildcrafted herbal products, including PetEssiance Herbal Pet Tea and Pet Tonic (Essiac formula with Cat's Claw and Astragalus), Pet Colon Comfort, and Well Pet Energy Essences.

Flower Essences

Spirit Essences Holistic Remedies for Animals
www.spiritessences.com
877-857-7474
Wonderful essence formulas for animals, including Peacemaker, Graceful Aging, Healthy Helper, Vaccine Detox, and Stress Stopper. Founded by Dr. Jean Hofve in 1995, Spirit Essences remains the only line of essence remedies formulated by a veterinarian.

Health Devices

BEMER International
818-707-6331
Physical vascular therapy device. (Distributed by Celestial Pets)

NanoVi (formerly Active Air) Device
818-707-6331
NanoVi bioidentical signaling device, FDA-registered Class I medical devices for improving cell metabolism and triggering the body's natural resistance to oxidative stress. (Distributed by Celestial Pets)

Feel-Rite Pet Products
866-928-9007

330-928-8000
www.magnamat.com
Manufacturers of the Magna-Mat line
of magnetic/orthopedic pet beds, pads,
and mats.

Lyon Technologies
888-LYON-USA
www.lyonusa.com
Distributors of Thermotex infrared heating pads and pet beds

Purple Plates
860-830-9069
www.purpleplates.com
Tesla's purple positive energy plates,
disks, and pet collars

Homeopathic Remedies

Capitol Drugs
818-905-8338
310-289-1125
800-819-9098
www.capitoldrugs.com
Alternative and traditional pharmacy
carrying homeopathic remedies, herbs,
vitamins, books, and more

Guna
888-486-2835

www.gunainc.com
The Guna method is a unique approach to homeopathic and biotherapeutic medicine

Heel (for practitioners)
  Heel/BHI (over-the-counter retail)
800-621-7644
505-293-3843
www.heelusa.com
Makers of Traumeel and other homeopathic formulas using combinations of key biotherapeutic ingredients (homotoxicology)

Natural Health Supply
888-689-1608
505-474-9175
www.a2zhomeopathy.com
Homeopathic remedies, kits, books, and supplies

Similasan Homeopathic Remedies
800-426-1644
www.similasanusa.com
Homeopathic eye drops

Nontoxic Cleaning and Pest Control

Fleabusters
800-666-3532

www.fleabusters.com
Distributors of Rx for Fleas Plus and
dust mite and yard products (beneficial
nematodes)

Pure Comfort Shampoos
Herbal shampoo containing essential oil
of Erigeron canadensis (Canadian fleabane) for the treatment of fleas. Herbal
shampoo without Erigeron also available. (Distributed by Celestial Pets)

Seventh Generation
800-456-1191
802-658-3773
www.seventhgeneration.com
Green cleaning and laundry products,
paper goods, baby and feminine products. Free e-newsletter and coupons
available.

Miscellaneous Products

Corning Incorporated
800-999-3436
www.pyrexware.com
Pyrex glass bowls with tight-fitting lids
to keep dog food very fresh

Himalayan Pure Crystal Salt Products
Lamps, candle holders, bath salts, and
table salt (Distributed by Celestial Pets)

LL's Magnetic Clay (topical magnesium)
www.magneticclay.com/174.html
Suppliers of Ancient Minerals, concentrated, ultrapure magnesium oil for topical use, and bath salts

Music for Pets and People
860-567-9217
www.musicforpetsandpeople.com

Yuk2e
301-299-9279
www.vetplanet.net
A safe, nontoxic but terrible-tasting gel to deter pets from licking wounds, lesions, splints, and IV catheters

Water Products

Multipure Drinking Water Systems
800-622-9206
702-360-8880
www.multipureco.com
Water filtration systems

Double Helix Water
www.doublehelixwater.com/
  #a_aid=Celestial_Pets
Ultra-pure stable water clusters (Distributed by Celestial Pets)

West Coast Water Filtration
800-834-2882
www.westcoastwaterfiltration.com
Nationwide installation of small and whole house water filtration systems

CAW Industries
605-343-8100
www.dr-willardswater.com
Willard Water (catalyst altered water, or CAW)

The employees of Thorndike Press hope you have enjoyed this Large Print book. All our Thorndike, Wheeler, and Kennebec Large Print titles are designed for easy reading, and all our books are made to last. Other Thorndike Press Large Print books are available at your library, through selected bookstores, or directly from us.

For information about titles, please call:
  (800) 223-1244

or visit our Web site at:
  http://gale.cengage.com/thorndike

To share your comments, please write:
  Publisher
  Thorndike Press
  10 Water St., Suite 310
  Waterville, ME 04901